Good Psychiatric Management *and* Dialectical Behavior Therapy

A Clinician's Guide to Integration and Stepped Care

Good Psychiatric Management *and* Dialectical Behavior Therapy

A Clinician's Guide to Integration and Stepped Care

Edited by

Anne K.I. Sonley, J.D., M.D., FRCPC

Lois W. Choi-Kain, M.D., M.Ed.

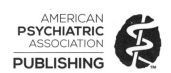

AMERICAN
PSYCHIATRIC
ASSOCIATION
PUBLISHING

If you wish to buy 50 or more copies of the same title, please go to www.appi.org/specialdiscounts for more information.

Copyright © 2021 American Psychiatric Association Publishing

ALL RIGHTS RESERVED

First Edition

Manufactured in the United States of America on acid-free paper
24 23 22 21 20   5 4 3 2 1

American Psychiatric Association Publishing
800 Maine Avenue SW, Suite 900
Washington, DC 20024-2812
www.appi.org

Library of Congress Cataloging-in-Publication Data
Names: Sonley, Anne K.I., editor. | Choi-Kain, Lois W., editor. | American Psychiatric Association Publishing, publisher.
Title: Good psychiatric management and dialectical behavior therapy : a clinician's guide to integration and stepped care / edited by Anne K.I. Sonley, Lois W. Choi-Kain
Description: First edition. | Washington, D.C. : American Psychatric Association Publishing, [2021] | Includes bibliographical references and index.
Identifiers: LCCN 2020035448 (print) | LCCN 2020035449 (ebook) | ISBN 9781615373413 (paperback ; alk. paper) | ISBN 9781615373727 (ebook)
Subjects: MESH: Borderline Personality Disorder—therapy | Dialectical Behavior Therapy—methods | Psychotherapy—methods | Case Management
Classification: LCC RC569.5.B67 (print) | LCC RC569.5.B67 (ebook) | NLM WM 190.5.B5 | DDC 616.85/852—dc23
LC record available at https://lccn.loc.gov/2020035448
LC ebook record available at https://lccn.loc.gov/2020035449

British Library Cataloguing in Publication Data
A CIP record is available from the British Library.

Contents

Lois W. Choi-Kain, M.D., M.Ed.
Anne K.I. Sonley, J.D., M.D., FRCPC

Lois W. Choi-Kain, M.D., M.Ed.
Anne K.I. Sonley, J.D., M.D., FRCPC

Anne K.I. Sonley, J.D., M.D., FRCPC
Lois W. Choi-Kain, M.D., M.Ed.

Lois W. Choi-Kain, M.D., M.Ed.
Evan Iliakis, B.A.
Gabrielle Ilagan, B.A.

Deanna Mercer, M.D., FRCPC
Anne K.I. Sonley, J.D., M.D., FRCPC
Lois W. Choi-Kain, M.D., M.Ed.

Contributors

Lois W. Choi-Kain, M.D., M.Ed.
Director, Gunderson Personality Disorders Institute, Belmont, Massachusetts; Assistant Professor of Psychiatry, Harvard Medical School, Boston, Massachusetts

Gabrielle Ilagan, B.A.
Clinical Research Assistant, Gunderson Personality Disorders Institute, McLean Hospital, Belmont, Massachusetts

Evan Iliakis, B.A.
Medical Student, Perelman School of Medicine, University of Pennsylvania, Philadelphia, Pennsylvania

Paul S. Links, M.D., M.Sc., FRCPC
Professor, Department of Psychiatry and Behavioural Neurosciences, McMaster University, Hamilton, Ontario, Canada

Shelley McMain, Ph.D., C.Psych.
Associate Professor and Director, Psychotherapy, Humanities, and Psychosocial Interventions (PHPI) Division, Department of Psychiatry, University of Toronto; Head, Borderline Personality Disorder Clinic, Centre for Addiction and Mental Health, Toronto, Ontario, Canada

Deanna Mercer, M.D., FRCPC
Assistant Professor, Department of Psychiatry, University of Ottawa; Borderline Personality Disorder Clinic, Canadian Mental Health Association, Ottawa, Ontario, Canada

Anne K.I. Sonley, J.D., M.D., FRCPC
Lecturer, University of Toronto; Psychiatrist, Borderline Personality Disorders Clinic, Centre for Addiction and Mental Health, Toronto, Ontario, Canada

Disclosure of Competing Interests

The following contributors to this book have indicated a financial interest in or other affiliation with a commercial supporter, a manufacturer of a commercial product, a provider of a commercial service, a nongovernmental organization, and/or a government agency, as listed below:

Lois W. Choi-Kain, M.D., M.Ed.—*Royalties:* American Psychiatric Association Publishing (author/coeditor); Harvard Continuing Education (course director); Springer (author/coeditor)

Paul S. Links, M.D., M.Sc., FRCPC—*Royalties:* American Psychiatric Association Publishing (for *Handbook of Good Psychiatric Management for Borderline Personality Disorder*)

The following contributors have indicated that they have no financial interests or other affiliations that represent or could appear to represent a competing interest with the contributions to this book:

Gabrielle Ilagan, B.A.

Evan Iliakis, B.A.

Shelley McMain, Ph.D., C.Psych.

Deanna Mercer, M.D., FRCPC

Anne K. I. Sonley, J.D., M.D., FRCPC

Acknowledgments

This book was born out of a lucky convergence of events during a difficult time. In the last book that John Gunderson and I (L.C.-K.) would develop together, *Applications of Good Psychiatric Management for Borderline Personality Disorder: A Practical Guide* (Choi-Kain and Gunderson 2019), we asked Deanna Mercer and Paul Links to join me in writing a chapter on the integration of good psychiatric management (GPM) with dialectical behavior therapy (DBT). It was only when we received the first draft, which was over 70 pages long, that we realized how substantial a project it was. Although we needed to revise the chapter significantly for the purposes of the *Practical Guide*, that first draft in its entirety was the basis of this book.

Anne Sonley was a senior resident at the University of Toronto at the time, working in Shelley McMain's DBT program at the Centre for Addiction and Mental Health. Shelley's DBT versus GPM trial had put GPM on the map. Anne inquired about doing an elective rotation with me at the Adult Borderline Center and Training Institute, now renamed the Gunderson Personality Disorders Institute. She landed in Boston for her 6-month research rotation in the summer of 2018, when we were immersed in the editing process of the *Practical Guide*. Given Anne's excellent training in DBT, she was assigned the DBT and GPM chapter with the formidable task of converting an excellent, comprehensive, and lengthy discussion of DBT's and GPM's overlaps into a chapter half that length. Her investment in that project was admirable, and even more so was her dedication to the idea of turning its original draft into this now completed book. Aside from the work Anne did with Deanna and Paul, whose contributions are the heart of this book, she also enlisted help from Shelley McMain to write a chapter called "Dialectical Behavior Therapy Tool Kit" (Chapter 5), which is among the best brief DBT resources I (L.C.-K.) have read. I am grateful to Anne for her work in bringing together two central figures in the DBT versus GPM trial, Shelley McMain and Paul Links, in this book with us and Deanna Mercer, to extend the applicability of GPM as well as DBT in abbreviated and boiled-down formats. Personally, I have enjoyed the opportunity to have supported

Anne's growth from the position of a student to a growing expert and collaborator in the mission to improve access to effective treatment both for patients with borderline personality disorder (BPD) and for the clinicians who want to do better for those patients. Anne's work is a testament to the fact that young professionals can move the field forward with their work, even at the beginning of their careers, with earnest dedication and good training.

I (A.S.) would like to start off by thanking Lois Choi-Kain, whose mentorship has made it possible for me to participate in this project and who welcomed me warmly in Boston when I was a Canadian away from home. I would also like to thank the clinicians and staff at the Gunderson Residence and McLean Hospital who allowed me to learn about BPD treatments in their setting. I would especially like to thank Evan, Gabs, Leila, Amanda, Lauren, Alex, Justin, and Kim, who were my family away from home in Boston. I would also like to personally thank Deanna Mercer, whose lengthy writing on the topic of integrating DBT and GPM inspired this book and whose lecture on personality disorders first inspired me to enter this field. I would like to thank my mentors in Toronto, Shelley McMain and Carmen Wiebe, as well as all of the clinicians in our clinic who have taught and continue to teach me how to provide good DBT. I would like to thank my current and former clients who have taught me and continue to teach me how to provide good DBT and good GPM. I would like to thank my friends/generalist clinicians who provided feedback on this book, especially Jacky, Courtney, Rayanne, Smrita, and Dorothy, and I would like to thank my partner Gil for reading and rereading this manuscript more times than any human should have to.

We both (L.C.-K. and A.S.) want to thank Evan Iliakis and Gabrielle (Gabs) Ilagan, who are by title research assistants, but in reality, they are major collaborators in all the work of the Gunderson Personality Disorders Institute. Evan and Gabs did a significant amount of editing, formatting, and streamlining of the final product. Their contributions and company have been enormously vital to both of us in completing this work.

Finally, we want to commemorate the late John G. Gunderson, whose dedication to the cause of improving care for patients with BPD and their families was boundless. We thank John for all the work he did to establish the BPD diagnosis and elucidate its symptoms, relationship to other psychiatric disorders, longitudinal course, genetics, and treatments. Specifically, John's efforts to disseminate GPM have increased access to care for people with chronic suicidal ideation and self-harm. Before he passed away, John noted that his idea of the afterlife was in all that he had left behind. John specifically named the trainees he taught over his lifetime as his legacy. It is in this book and our GPM efforts that we keep Gunderson's dedicated spirit alive to continue to do better for those with BPD, proving they are people who can get better and that all mental health professionals can help them in doing so.

Lois W. Choi-Kain, M.D., M.Ed.
Anne K.I. Sonley, J.D., M.D., FRCPC

Reference

Choi-Kain LW, Gunderson JG (eds): Applications of Good Psychiatric Management for Borderline Personality Disorder: A Practical Guide. Washington, DC, American Psychiatric Association Publishing, 2019

Introduction

Lois W. Choi-Kain, M.D., M.Ed.

Anne K.I. Sonley, J.D., M.D., FRCPC

Treatment for BPD: What Works

Treatment options for borderline personality disorder (BPD) have vastly improved over the last three decades with the development of evidence-based psychotherapies. Dialectical behavior therapy (DBT; Linehan 1993) was the first of these modern treatments to bring new hope that BPD—with its concerning and complex profile of emotion dysregulation, self-harm and suicidal behaviors, impulsivity, and interpersonal instability—could in fact be treated effectively. Given BPD's morbidity and mortality and lack of consistent improvement with standard treatment, clinicians have been understandably hesitant to treat these patients. With the advent of manualized empirically validated treatments that are specially tailored to treat the problems of BPD, optimism about clinical interventions for this group of suffering individuals has increased considerably.

In addition to DBT, multiple evidence-based treatments, such as mentalization-based treatment (MBT; Bateman and Fonagy 1999, 2009), transference-focused psychotherapy (Clarkin et al. 2007; Doering et al. 2010), and schema-focused therapy (Giesen-Bloo et al. 2006), have been added to the tool kit of effective therapies for BPD. These treatments significantly reduce self-harm and suicidal behaviors and reduce health care utilization. They are also cost-effective, with average cost savings of $2,987.82 per patient per year (Meuldijk et al. 2017). Experts in the field have attempted to identify common factors among these varied evidence-based treatments that contribute to their efficacy. Glen Gabbard has posed the essential question: "Could it be that any thoughtful, systematic approach to borderline personality disorder, based on our knowledge of the disorder, is potentially helpful, whatever its theoretical underpinnings or technical approach?" (Gabbard 2007, p. 854).

What appears central to these treatments that work are six core features (Bateman 2012; Sledge et al. 2014; Weinberg et al. 2011). First, a clear treatment framework, outlined in a structured manual, provides a clinical map for professionals and patients alike, with clear recommendations for common predictable problems, so that treatment is guided by rational recommendations rather than in-the-moment reactions to stressful situations. Second, a model of psychopathology that is carefully explained allows the clinician and patient to understand the problems their treatment aims to address. Third, a focus on emotion processing allows the patient to learn how their actions arise from reactions to feelings. Fourth, evidence-based treatments for BPD place agency for change within the patient to encourage patient proactivity, rather than dependency on the clinician to know all the answers and provide solutions. Fifth, an active stance by the clinician focuses on the here and now and often involves self-disclosure of the clinician's internal experience. Sixth, all treatments proven effective for BPD focus on the treatment relationship, employing empathic validation, and a collaborative stance, which is important given the interpersonal difficulties inherent to the disorder.

The good news is that the range of options has greatly expanded for clinicians and their patients with BPD. The bad news is that these specialized treatments remain difficult to access because of the limited number of professionals who are able to provide them (Iliakis et al. 2019). Although these specialized therapies work for BPD, they also require a significant amount of training, supervision, and time to learn and implement (Choi-Kain et al. 2016; Iliakis et al. 2019). The survival of specialized BPD programs in real-world settings is challenged by high costs and difficulties with staff retention and maintenance of institutional support (Bales et al. 2017; King et al. 2018; Swales et al. 2012). BPD is prevalent in most clinical settings, but the clinicians best trained to treat BPD remain limited in number and are difficult to access because of waitlists. In reality, specialized BPD treatments are rarely available as immediate dispositions from emergency rooms, inpatient hospitalizations, or primary care referrals. Are less intensive treatments available that can still provide appropriate care to individuals with BPD? Given limited access to specialized evidence-based treatments for BPD, efforts to increase the availability of effective treatment are needed.

Generalist clinical management approaches for BPD meet this need for more accessible care. After it became known that the specialized manualized psychotherapies for BPD outperformed "treatment as usual" or "waitlist" conditions in randomized controlled trials, researchers felt that trials involving more robust comparator treatments were needed to test whether the efficacy of the specialized treatments resulted from their specific approach and techniques. Two of the largest, most scientifically rigorous randomized controlled trials of outpatient psychotherapies for BPD compared general clinical management approaches with specialized BPD treatments—that is, DBT and MBT. The generalist approaches in these trials were built by BPD experts who trained clinicians using manualized national guidelines (American Psychiatric Association 2001; National Institute for Health and Care Excellence 2009) and incorporated psychotherapeutic elements but did not rely on the contents or techniques associated with the specialized treatments.

In Canada, Shelley McMain's research team reported that 1 year of general psychiatric management (GPM) for treating patients with BPD performed as well as DBT at posttreatment and at 2-year follow-up (McMain et al. 2009, 2012). In this study, DBT was provided in a standard format, with weekly individual therapy, weekly group therapy, availability of 24-hour coaching, and weekly clinician meetings. In contrast, GPM involved weekly individual therapy and weekly clinician meetings. The absence of difference in outcomes was surprising given the expectation that DBT would outperform GPM. Similarly, in the United Kingdom, Anthony Bateman and Peter Fonagy reported that people with BPD improved significantly with both "structured clinical management" and MBT; of note, however, patients with comorbid personality disorders in addition to BPD did better with MBT than with structured clinical management (Bateman and Fonagy 2009, 2013).

Generalist approaches to BPD care, such as GPM, open new horizons to expanding care options so that more mental health professionals can be sufficiently educated to treat people with BPD. However, the availability of such generalist approaches does not mean that specialized evidence-based treatments should not be used; rather, specialized treatments, as scarce and more intensive resources, might be better reserved for specific populations. Treatment for BPD is not one size fits all and could be scaled for different clinical stages, situations, settings, and levels of motivation or readiness to do intensive psychotherapy. In this manual, we provide a framework for implementing a stepped care model in settings where access to specialized treatments is limited. We suggest that the principles of GPM are a basic foundation that all clinicians can learn and that GPM might be implemented within a stepped care model as a precursor to a more specialized treatment, such as DBT; in combination with a DBT skills–only group; as a step down from DBT; or as a plan B in cases in which DBT does not seem to be effective or the patient lacks readiness.

GPM and DBT: Combining What Works

Given what we know about generalist treatments for BPD and what we know about the common factors that are effective in treating BPD, we also propose in this book a framework for how one might go about providing care to patients with BPD in settings where standardized evidence-based treatments such as DBT and MBT are limited or not available. In this book, we are prioritizing pragmatism by suggesting what works in terms of reasonable evidence, pragmatic allocation of public health resources, and real-world clinical experience implementing evidence-based treatments for BPD.

This manual draws on GPM, a generalist model, and integrates principles drawn from DBT, a specialist treatment. GPM is an approach to treating BPD that requires minimal training (see Appendix E), is flexible, and is feasible for generalists to learn and use. We also present boiled-down essential concepts and tools from DBT, which has the most robust evidence base of all the treatments that work for BPD (Stoffers et al. 2012). DBT represents a gold standard for BPD treatment; however, its encyclopedic content is often not accessible to generalist clinicians. We feel that this combination of GPM, which every clinician can learn, and a focused set of techniques from DBT provides a useful blend of the best of generalist and specialist tools for clinicians to use.

In this clinician's guide, we start in Chapter 1 with a brief overview of both GPM and DBT, providing broad strokes about how BPD is conceptualized in each model. The second chapter introduces the idea of a stepped care model for BPD, which proposes briefer, less intensive, and less specialized approaches to managing patients, depending on clinical stage, interest, and available resources. Chapter 2, on stepped care, provides a menu of ways clinicians and programs can use GPM, DBT, and any other specialist psychotherapy for BPD. In Chapters 3 and 4, the common principles found in both DBT and GPM are reviewed. These are principles that any generalist clinician can incorporate into their practice, including clinician stance, treatment organization, and an approach to managing crises. Techniques specific to each treatment are then described in greater detail in Chapters 5 and 6, the DBT and GPM tool kits. These tool kits summarize the top skills and techniques from each treatment for clinicians who are interested in using them in their practice. Chapter 7 includes a full set of case illustrations that show the application of DBT and GPM in common clinical scenarios. These vignettes demonstrate how DBT and GPM can be integrated into primary care settings, emergency rooms, and generalist mental health settings where specialized psychotherapies for BPD are either not available or not well suited. The clinicians in the vignettes are often residents in psychiatry or generalists without access to immediate referrals to DBT, or even to psychiatry, because in most regions appointments with psychiatry services are severely limited. Chapter 8 concludes the book with an integrative summary of the key points that clinicians can use to understand patients with BPD and manage their care.

This book is aimed at general psychiatrists, social workers, mental health nurses, psychiatry residents, family physicians, psychologists, and other mental health clinicians who practice in communities where evidence-based treatments for BPD are difficult to access. For some professionals, practicing a specialized evidence-based psychotherapy for BPD in its pure form is not compatible with their clinical context, level of interest, or access to supervision. This guide introduces concepts, techniques, and tools for working with patients with BPD. It is not an exhaustive discourse on DBT or GPM but is meant to provide an accessible overview of how one could provide treatment incorporating GPM and DBT in either an integrated or stepped care way. Our hope is that this manual will provide some guidance to generalist mental health clinicians to provide "good enough" care to patients with BPD, many of whom are currently struggling to access any care at all. In the words of BPD expert John Gunderson, "If you know enough to avoid being harmful, you can be, surprisingly, very helpful" (Gunderson and Links 2014, p. 4).

References

American Psychiatric Association: Practice guideline for the treatment of patients with borderline personality disorder. Am J Psychiatry 158 (10 suppl):1–52, 2001

Bales DL, Verheul R, Hutsebaut J: Barriers and facilitators to the implementation of mentalization-based treatment (MBT) for borderline personality disorder. Pers Ment Health 11:118–131, 2017

Bateman AW: Treating borderline personality disorder in clinical practice. Am J Psychiatry 169(6):560–563, 2012

Bateman A, Fonagy P: Effectiveness of partial hospitalization in the treatment of borderline personality disorder: a randomized controlled trial. Am J Psychiatry 156(10):1563–1569, 1999

Bateman A, Fonagy P: Randomized controlled trial of outpatient mentalization-based treatment versus structured clinical management for borderline personality disorder. Am J Psychiatry 166(12):1355–1364, 2009

Bateman A, Fonagy P: Impact of clinical severity on outcomes of mentalisation-based treatment for borderline personality disorder. Br J Psychiatry. 203(3):221–227, 2013

Choi-Kain LW, Albert EB, Gunderson JG: Evidence-based treatments for borderline personality disorder: implementation, integration, and stepped care. Harv Rev Psychiatry 24(5):342–356, 2016

Clarkin JF, Levy KN, Lenzenweger MF, Kernberg OF: Evaluating three treatments for borderline personality disorder: a multiwave study. Am J Psychiatry 164(6):922–928, 2007

Doering S, Hörz S, Rentrop M, et al: Transference-focused psychotherapy v. treatment by community psychotherapists for borderline personality disorder: randomised controlled trial. Br J Psychiatry 196(5):389–395, 2010

Gabbard GO: Do all roads lead to Rome? New findings on borderline personality disorder. Am J Psychiatry 164(6):853–855, 2007

Giesen-Bloo J, van Dyck R, Spinhoven P, et al: Outpatient psychotherapy for borderline personality disorder: randomized trial of schema-focused therapy vs transference-focused psychotherapy. Arch Gen Psychiatry 63(6):649–658, 2006

Gunderson JG, Links P: Handbook of Good Psychiatric Management for Borderline Personality Disorder. Washington, DC, American Psychiatric Publishing, 2014

Iliakis EA, Sonley AKI, Ilagan GS, Choi-Kain LW: Treatment of borderline personality disorder: is supply adequate to meet public health needs? Psychiatr Serv 70(9):772–781, 2019

King JC, Hibbs R, Saville CWN, Swales MA: The survivability of dialectical behavior therapy programmes: a mixed methods analysis of barriers and facilitators to implementation within UK healthcare settings. BMC Psychiatry 18(1):302, 2018

Landes SJ, Rodriguez AL, Smith BN, et al: Barriers, facilitators, and benefits of implementation of dialectical behavior therapy in routine care: results from a national program evaluation survey in the Veterans Health Administration. Transl Behav Med 7(4):832–844, 2017

Linehan MM: Cognitive-Behavioral Treatment of Borderline Personality Disorder. New York, Guilford, 1993

McMain SF, Links PS, Gnam WH, et al: A randomized trial of dialectical behavior therapy versus general psychiatric management for borderline personality disorder. Am J Psychiatry 166(12):1365–1374, 2009

McMain SF, Guimond T, Streiner DL, et al: Dialectical behavior therapy compared with general psychiatric management for borderline personality disorder: clinical outcomes and functioning over a 2-year follow-up. Am J Psychiatry 169(6):650–661, 2012

Meuldijk D, McCarthy A, Bourke ME, Grenyer BFS: The value of psychological treatment for borderline personality disorder: systematic review and cost offset analysis of economic evaluations. PLoS One 12(3):e0151592, 2017

National Institute for Health and Care Excellence: Borderline Personality Disorder: Treatment and Management (Report No CG78). London, National Institute for Health and Care Excellence, 2009

Sledge W, Plakun EM, Bauer S, et al: Psychotherapy for suicidal patients with borderline personality disorder: an expert consensus review of common factors across five therapies. Borderline Personal Disord Emot Dysregul 1:16, 2014

Stoffers JM, Völlm BA, Rücker G, et al: Psychological therapies for people with borderline personality disorder. Cochrane Database Syst Rev (8):CD005652, 2012

Swales MA, Taylor B, Hibbs RA: Implementing dialectical behavior therapy: programme survival in routine healthcare settings. J Ment Health 21(6):548–555, 2012

Weinberg I, Ronningstam E, Goldblatt MJ, et al: Common factors in empirically supported treatments of borderline personality disorder. Curr Psychiatry Rep 13(1):60–68, 2011

1

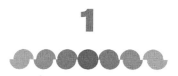

A Brief Overview of Good Psychiatric Management and Dialectical Behavior Therapy

Anne K.I. Sonley, J.D., M.D., FRCPC

Lois W. Choi-Kain, M.D., M.Ed.

This chapter provides an introduction to the theory, general principles, goals, and structure of good psychiatric management (GPM) and dialectical behavior therapy (DBT). The chapter ends by underscoring the compatibility of the two approaches and providing examples of how they can work together to inform treatment.

Overview of Good Psychiatric Management

General psychiatric management, or "good psychiatric management" as it was rebranded by John Gunderson, is a principle-driven approach well suited for generalist clinicians treating people with borderline personality disorder (BPD). At its core, GPM relies on fundamental clinical tasks, such as diagnostic disclosure, psychoeducation, and enhancing accountability, to work on reducing and managing BPD symptoms. It additionally provides a theoretical model for understanding, and thereby managing, the symptoms of BPD.

GPM proposes that people with BPD are born with a genetic predisposition to be interpersonally hypersensitive. As a result, people with BPD develop a characteristic interpersonal pattern that can get in the way of building stable interpersonal relationships and can also get in the way of other functional goals related to work and school. This prototypical pattern is illustrated in Figure 1–1.

When patients with BPD feel connected to others, they are less symptomatic, more effective, and more open to learning, but they also tend to idealize others and are anxiously vigilant for signs of rejection. When they begin feeling interpersonally threatened because of real or perceived rejection, they may start to become angry or devalue others, and their symptoms become more evident. At this point, they are still engaged, albeit angrily. If the patient receives support from others while feeling interpersonally threatened, the patient then returns to the "connected" state. However, if other people withdraw in reaction to the patient's angry devaluation, this can then lead to increased distress, self-harm, paranoia, dissociation, and impulsive behaviors such as substance use, disordered eating, spending sprees, risky sexual activity, or reckless driving. At this point in the symptomatic cycle, it is difficult to intervene collaboratively, as the person with BPD becomes more difficult to reach through words. If left alone without the containment of a relationship, the patient may descend into hopelessness and suicidal behavior. Often at this point others, including clinicians, family, or friends, might act unilaterally by putting the patient in a safe setting (i.e., in a hospital or on suicide watch). The patient can then reconstitute into a connected state; however, this brings the cycle into a position where others are central to solving problems of safety, a situation that ultimately reinforces problematic dependencies.

The clinician can interrupt this pattern in several ways. One way is to help the patient become aware of the pattern and notice common interpersonal stressors. The clinician and patient can work together to try to intervene when the patient is feeling threatened earlier in the symptom cycle, before the patient begins acting impulsively or feeling hopeless and suicidal. Intervention earlier in the descent toward reckless action or despairing suicidality is crucial because it allows the clinician and patient to collaborate on efforts to understand and problem solve more effectively. The GPM clinician advises the patient to be prepared for inevitable moments of feeling threatened. Together, the GPM clinician and the patient with BPD reduce the likelihood of intolerable loneliness by acting in more prosocial ways that make others want to be with them and by broadening their support system so they are less affected

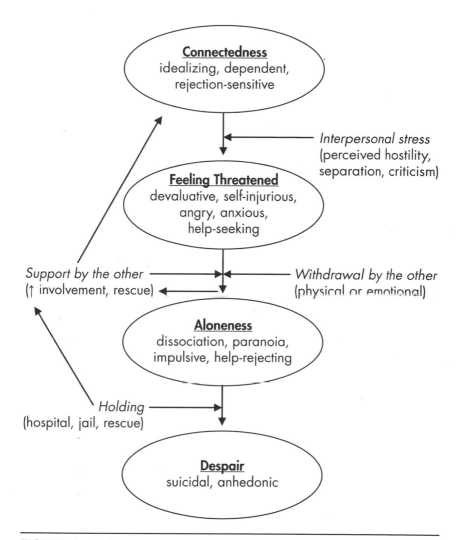

FIGURE 1–1.   Interpersonal coherence model of borderline personality disorder.

Source.   Reprinted from Gunderson JG, Links P: *Handbook of Good Psychiatric Management for Borderline Personality Disorder*. Washington, DC, American Psychiatric Association, 2014, p. 14. Copyright © 2014 American Psychiatric Publishing. Used with permission.

by ups and downs in intense exclusive relationships (e.g., romantic relationships). Self-reliance and reduced dependency on others are encouraged as they can serve as a buffer to the way others' reactions affect the person with BPD.

In addition to noticing these patterns, the clinician also builds a therapeutic alliance with the patient in which the patient feels connected to the clinician. This therapeutic alliance is enhanced by the clinician's frank feedback and consistent, responsive, and curious attitude toward the patient. Through the experience of consistently maintaining a reliable "good enough" connection with the clinician, sustained through both appreciative connected and angry devaluing states, the patient's sense of who they are can become more stable and coherent. Because of this integrated appreciation of these two sides of the person with BPD, the clinician provides at least one relationship that can serve as a "corrective experience" for the patient, one in which the patient experiences being heard and understood, balanced with reasonable expectations of being responsible for themselves and acting in a way that influences others to want to be around them.

The goals of treatment in GPM are to decrease subjective distress and BPD symptoms, while improving social functioning and interpersonal relationships. These are consistent with the general aims of any psychiatric treatment. The structure of GPM is flexible. It generally involves the patient and clinician meeting once per week, depending on the patient's needs and the clinician's availability. Attendance by the patient at any type of group available in the community is encouraged. Clinicians are advised to address their intersession availability with patients, and some phone access to the clinician between appointments is recommended, but dependency for safety is regarded with skepticism. Last, clinicians are strongly encouraged to have access to consultation with other clinicians (Gunderson and Links 2014).

Important elements of GPM include collaboratively providing the patient with a diagnosis and psychoeducation about BPD. In session, clinicians take an active role and focus on the patient's life outside of therapy. They encourage verbal discussion of the patient's feelings and interactions with others to stress thinking before acting. GPM emphasizes working with the patient to build a life for themselves and specifies that patients should focus on career and friends first, then romantic partners. GPM also provides guidance regarding managing comorbidities, medications, suicidal behavior and self-harm, hospitalization, working with multiple providers, working with families, and monitoring progress in treatment.

Overview of Dialectical Behavior Therapy

DBT is a manualized therapy designed to treat people with suicidal and self-harming behaviors. It has been studied in many randomized controlled trials and has one of the strongest evidence bases among BPD treatments (Stoffers et al. 2012). In DBT, the explanatory model of BPD focuses on emotional dysregulation as the core difficulty causing symptoms of BPD.

The biosocial model in DBT states that people with BPD are naturally more emotionally intense and sensitive. Furthermore, they return to their emotional baseline more slowly than the general population. Like most natural phenomena, emotional reactivity is thought to exist on a spectrum, with some individuals being more emotionally reactive, others being less emotionally reactive, and most being somewhere in the middle.

Being emotionally intense is not necessarily problematic in itself. There are many emotionally intense people who lead satisfying productive lives. The problem occurs when emotionally intense people grow up in an environment that may not be the best fit for them and they lack skills to manage that mismatch. For example, if an emotionally intense child grows up with parents and siblings who are not as emotionally intense as the child, these family members might not understand the child's emotional reactions very well and therefore might be prone to respond to the child in a way that intensifies rather than soothes negative emotions.

For instance, when watching a sad movie, other children in a family might be somewhat sad, whereas the emotionally intense child might start crying and take a long time to stop. Parents might naturally say, for example, "It's only a movie. Don't worry, calm down. Stop crying so much." Though reasonable, this attempt at emotional support actually conveys to the child that the child's response is abnormal and that the parent does not understand the child's emotional experience. In DBT, responses that convey a lack of understanding of someone's experience are called "invalidating" responses. In the above example, a more "validating" response might be to hug the child and say, "I know, it's a sad movie, right?"

DBT proposes that when emotionally intense people are exposed to repeated invalidation or to severe forms of invalidation, such as abuse or neglect, they can develop core symptoms of BPD. Repeated invalidation of a person's experience can lead the individual to start questioning their own judgment and emotional experience. This inability to trust one's own experience can lead to one of the core features of BPD:

an unstable sense of self. In an invalidating environment, individuals also have more difficulty learning to regulate their emotions, leading to further emotional dysregulation. This is often followed by the development of problematic coping behaviors such as self-harm, substance use, binge-eating behaviors, reckless driving, and other risky behaviors. It is not surprising that with the combination of an unstable sense of self and emotional dysregulation, individuals with BPD frequently have unstable interpersonal relationships. High levels of emotional dysregulation and difficulties with sense of self may also result in dissociation and paranoia in stressful situations. DBT involves learning skills that enable individuals to better manage emotional intensity and emotional dysregulation. Management of invalidation is also introduced and explicitly addressed within the treatment.

When initially developing DBT, Marsha Linehan first used cognitive-behavioral therapy (CBT) type techniques with suicidal patients, such as teaching them effective problem-solving strategies (Linehan and Wilks 2015). This approach was experienced as quite invalidating and resulted in clients becoming angry with therapists and dropping out of treatment. She then tried a therapeutic approach that focused mostly on validating the patient's experience, similar to Rogerian person-centered therapy. Although patients felt understood, steps toward reducing self-harm and building a life worth living did not occur. The synthesis of these two approaches resulted in DBT, which incorporates both change-oriented strategies, such as those seen in CBT, and validating acceptance strategies, such as those seen in person-centered therapy. This synthesis balances understanding with accountability for change in a way that seems to work particularly well in helping people with BPD to build a life worth living and to stop engaging in self-harm behaviors.

What is dialectical about DBT? A dialectic involves two opposing poles that may appear to be incompatible with each other but are both true at the same time. Awareness of these poles can provide a more comprehensive perspective, and sometimes the poles can come together, resulting in a synthesis. As alluded to above, the key dialectic in DBT is that of acceptance and change. For example, DBT posits that people with BPD are doing the best that they can (acceptance). It also posits that they can do better (change). Although these two things appear to be in opposition, both can in fact be true at the same time and can come together in a synthesis: People with BPD are doing the best they can, and they can do better (Linehan 1993, pp. 106–108). Understanding the concept of dialectics can be useful to reduce all-or-nothing, black-and-white thinking, which is common in BPD.

Similar to GPM, the main goal of treatment in DBT is to help the patient build a life worth living. To help the patient attain this goal, DBT prioritizes intermediate goals, including stopping self-harm and suicidal behaviors, reducing behaviors that interfere with effective participation in therapy (e.g., nonattendance, lateness), and stopping other behaviors that the patient finds diminish their quality of life (e.g., substance use, binge eating). Standard DBT consists of 1 year of weekly individual therapy, weekly skills group training, after-hours skills coaching, and a therapist consultation group. DBT involves providing psychoeducation about the diagnosis as well as helping the patient identify prompting events and reinforcers of unwanted behaviors. It involves active problem solving and troubleshooting around different ways to change behavior. Finally, DBT involves learning skills to respond more effectively in situations that provoke strong emotion. Throughout therapy, the clinician's stance remains grounded in the dialectic of acceptance and change.

Integrating Principles From the Two Approaches

The theories of BPD proposed by DBT and GPM are not incompatible. DBT focuses on the broader concept of emotional dysregulation. In DBT, clinicians work with the patient to identify antecedents leading to dysregulation, which then leads to behavior that the patient considers problematic. The patient and clinician then use collaborative problem solving to identify ways the patient could respond more effectively next time. GPM highlights that one of the common sources of distress for people with BPD is difficulties in relationships, so when a clinician is working with a patient to determine what preceded distress and BPD symptoms, it is useful to consider the possibility of an interpersonal event. In addition, using GPM's interpersonal model to highlight common patterns can be helpful for patients. For example, by highlighting that many people who are interpersonally sensitive find that they feel threatened when faced with perceived interpersonal rejection, the clinician can help to normalize this reaction for patients and to mark this as something to focus on in treatment. When a patient notices anger, anxiety, or an urge to self-harm, they might then contemplate whether there was a perceived rejection or whether some other type of event has triggered this shift. The patient can then choose how to proceed, possibly using skills to react effectively in a way that is consistent with their values and goals. In this way, the underlying theories of DBT and GPM can work together quite well to inform treatment.

Key Points

- GPM proposes that people with BPD are naturally more interpersonally sensitive and that incidents of interpersonal rejection or hostility are often what prompt BPD symptoms to manifest.

- DBT proposes that people with BPD are naturally more emotionally intense and that repeated invalidation of their emotions and lack of skills for managing this emotional intensity leads to BPD symptoms.

- GPM encourages providing the patient with psychoeducation about BPD, helping the patient make connections between interpersonal stress and symptoms, and taking a stance of curiosity and understanding to develop the therapeutic alliance.

- DBT involves balancing change-oriented strategies (teaching skills and problem-solving) with acceptance-oriented strategies (increasing understanding of the person's emotions and behaviors as valid).

- Both GPM and DBT encourage "building a life worth living" as a goal of treatment, which often involves reducing maladaptive coping behaviors and increasing social and interpersonal functioning.

- GPM involves individual sessions (frequency is flexible) and recommends patient involvement in any type of group, as well as therapist consultation with other clinicians who treat BPD.

- Standard DBT involves weekly individual sessions, weekly group skills training, between-session skills training, and a weekly therapist consultation group.

———————— ●●● ————————

References

Gunderson JG, Links P: Handbook of Good Psychiatric Management for Borderline Personality Disorder. Washington DC: American Psychiatric Association, 2014

Linehan MM: Cognitive-Behavioral Treatment of Borderline Personality Disorder. New York, Guilford, 1993

Linehan MM, Wilks CR: The course and evolution of dialectical behavior therapy. Am J Psychother 69(2):97–110, 2015

Stoffers JM, Völlm BA, Rücker G, et al: Psychological therapies for people with borderline personality disorder. Cochrane Database Syst Rev 8:CD005652, 2012

2

●●●●●●●

Integration of Good Psychiatric Management and Dialectical Behavior Therapy With Stepped Care for Borderline Personality Disorder

Lois W. Choi-Kain, M.D., M.Ed.

Evan Iliakis, B.A.

Gabrielle Ilagan, B.A.

The rise of evidence-based treatments for borderline personality disorder (BPD) has powerfully reversed the stigma associated with the diagnosis, bringing hope that patients with BPD can get better with good clinical care (Choi-Kain et al. 2017a, 2017b). Among these treatments, dialectical behavior therapy (DBT) is the most extensively studied, with efficacy proven across several trials (Cristea et al. 2017; Stoffers et al. 2012). Its extensive training requirements, costs, and multimodality (Brodsky and Stanley 2013; Iliakis et al. 2019) ensure that patients receive high-quality care, although access is limited (Iliakis et al. 2019).

Various levels of care, from brief psychoeducational interventions to lengthier specialized treatments such as DBT, have places in the armamentarium of treatments for BPD. Different clinical environments, the clinicians staffing them, and the patients visiting various levels of care require different interventions. An assumption that any specific lengthy outpatient psychotherapy approach is the solution in all cases, regardless of setting, patient preferences, and access to care, is short-sighted. Stepped care models organize different intensities of care and also create pathways of intermediate levels of care so that the step-down from emergency room or inpatient level of care to outpatient care is not more drastic than either the patient or clinician can manage. Various stepped care models that emphasize brief care, less intensive preventive interventions, and lower levels of longer-term maintenance have been proposed. These models consider shorter-term versus longer-term care, clinical staging, responsiveness and motivation for treatment, step-downs from acute states, and gateways to longer-term treatment if desired and needed. In this chapter, we review these various stepped care options as possible ways in which different care settings can organize and triage care for patients with BPD. Table 2–1 summarizes the models in the order in which they are discussed in the chapter, starting with three conceptual models, followed by two empirically tested and implemented models.

Stepped Care Models for Borderline Personality Disorder

Brief Versus Extended Care

First to propose a stepped care model, Joel Paris has long advocated for proper access to treatment for patients with BPD. Paris (2013) argues as well that lengthy and intensive psychotherapies create serious problems for health care access. As a result, a significant number of patients stay on waitlists or cannot find affordable care in the times of greatest need. Consequently, too many patients enter the system in crisis, seeking intensive levels of care, including emergency room visits and inpatient hospitalization, which are known to be potentially harmful for the longer-term course of BPD (Gunderson and Links 2008; Knight 1953; Quaytman and Sharfstein 1997). Paris's stepped care model emphasizes brief treatment for the majority of patients, reserving extended treatment only for patients who fail to improve with a brief intervention and intermittent follow-up or for those who relapse. Paris (2017) emphasizes flexible triaging in terms of intensity and duration of care on a case-by-case basis.

TABLE 2–1.   Summary of stepped care models

Model	Steps of care and evidence	Rationale
Brief (12 weeks) vs. extended care (6–24 months) model (Paris 2013)	*Steps:* Brief treatment for most, step up if no improvement Extended treatment from outset for severe cases *Evidence:* Laporte et al. (2018) Of those completing brief treatment, only 12% requested/were referred to more treatment Significant improvements across outcomes in both groups	Efficiently allocates resources—reduces burden on specialist treatment centers, providing flexible options for patient preferences and clinical recommendations
Clinical staging model for youth with BPD and mood disorders (Chanen et al. 2016)	*Steps:* 1. Mild symptoms: psychoeducation, problem solving 2. First episode: brief generalist treatment, case management 3. Recurrence: medication, psychosocial strategies, specialized treatment 4. Persistent, unremitting symptoms: specialized treatment, clozapine, social participation in spite of disability	Provides a medical model of adjusting intervention to clinical severity and preventive care; offers less, more general support and advisement earlier; can provide more only if needed later; offers early intervention, reducing risk for later adverse outcomes

TABLE 2–1.   Summary of stepped care models (*continued*)

Model	Steps of care and evidence	Rationale
Clinical staging using evidence-based treatments for BPD (Choi-Kain et al. 2016)	*Steps:* 1. Subthreshold: psychoeducation 2. First episode: GPM psychoeducation, case management 3. Sustained threshold: GPM, medications, specialist groups 4. Remitting and relapsing: GPM and higher level of care or specialist treatment 5. Unremitting symptoms: low-frequency GPM, case management, supportive treatment	Provides a medical model of adjusting intervention to clinical severity and preventive care; accounts for patient motivation and inaccessibility of specialist treatment; focuses on pragmatic, not idealized, options

TABLE 2–1.　Summary of stepped care models *(continued)*

Model	Steps of care and evidence	Rationale
10-session GPM (assessment or treatment) as a gateway to determining further care (Kramer et al. 2011)	*Steps:* GPM for full assessment, diagnosis, and/or brief treatment 10-session assessment to determine need and plan for further specialist treatment *Evidence:* Kramer et al. (2014, 2017) 10-session GPM—medium-to-large effects on symptoms and interpersonal functioning Maintained over 6-month follow-up period Penzenstadler et al. (2018) Higher reduction in BPD symptoms in BPD+SUD group than in BPD group	Allows standardized start for treatment with diagnostic evaluation, psychoeducation, and goal setting; in itself, can help patients orient to their problems and what needs to change; can offer more treatment if available and desired by patient

TABLE 2–1.   Summary of stepped care models (continued)

Model	Steps of care and evidence	Rationale
Whole of service stepped care approach (Grenyer et al. 2018)	*Steps:* In four sessions over 4 weeks, implemented in outpatient stepped care clinics: Chain analysis of crisis Care plan Caregiver plan *Evidence:* Grenyer et al. (2018) Shorter hospital stays, fewer emergency room visits, cost savings Huxley et al. (2019) Only 14% stepped up to inpatient care Only 43% needed outpatient referrals	Facilitates step-down; prevents readmission; provides needed bridge between the intensive levels of care such as emergency rooms or hospitalization to outpatient care (For some patients) Adequately stabilizes if further care is not pursued

Note.   BPD=borderline personality disorder; GPM=good psychiatric management; SUD=substance use disorder.

Paris and his collaborators tested this pragmatic stepped care approach in a naturalistic study that followed 681 patients with BPD (Laporte et al. 2018). After an initial evaluation, most patients (86%) were referred to short-term treatment involving both individual and group therapy over 12 weeks, and a minority were referred to extended treatment lasting 6–24 months. The short-term treatment had a dropout rate comparable to that of other clinical trials of BPD (29%). Of those who completed the short-term treatment, only 12% requested or were referred to more treatment. Patients in both short-term and extended treatments showed significant improvements in self-reported measures of impulsivity, self-esteem, depression, emotional dysregulation, social adjustment, self-harm, and suicide attempts following treatment, but only those in the extended treatment showed statistically decreased drug and alcohol use. Patients in the extended care group improved significantly regardless of treatment length (6–12 months or 18–24 months). These findings suggest 1) that most patients can improve with short-term treatment and 2) that longer treatment does not necessarily produce more change, except in outcomes related to substance use. Notably, no single evidence-based manualized model was used, but elements of a number of effective treatments were eclectically employed with a team-based approach directed by experienced and expert leadership.

This brief care model provides the option to treat many more patients by limiting the length of treatment. If four-fifths of all patients received 3 months instead of 1 year of treatment, then a program using this model can accommodate approximately three times as many patients. It also accounts for the possibility that many patients do not need or want lengthier treatments. As Paris (2013) proposes, any clinical setting providing shorter-term treatment for BPD can serve more patients at a time of increased acuity. These patients can then receive more definitive BPD-focused care instead of containment through an emergency room or inpatient stay, which is costly and often leads to polypharmacy or interruption of important life responsibilities.

Clinical Staging Model for Early Intervention

Andrew Chanen and colleagues (2016) built a stepped care model of psychiatric treatment for youth using clinical staging to guide decision making (Table 2–2) (Chanen et al. 2016). Like other algorithms of medical decision making, this model implements the simple idea that intensity of care should increase with clinical staging. This framework allows for earlier intervention, reserving specialized and extended treatments for greater levels of clinical severity. Chanen and colleagues (2016) note

TABLE 2–2.   A potential clinical-staging model for bipolar disorder and borderline personality disorder

Clinical stage	Definition	Potential interventions
0	Increased risk of severe mood disorder or borderline personality disorder (e.g., family history, exposure to abuse or neglect, substance use) No specific current symptoms	Mental health literacy Self-help
1a	Mild or nonspecific symptoms of mood disorder or borderline personality disorder (e.g., disturbances in attention, emotion regulation, and behavior)	Formal mental health literacy; family psychoeducation, parenting skills; substance abuse reduction; supportive counseling/problem solving
1b	Subthreshold features of mood disorder or borderline personality disorder	Stage 1a interventions plus phase-specific psychosocial intervention (e.g., cognitive-behavioral therapy, HYPE early intervention for borderline personality disorder)
2	First episode of threshold mood disorder or borderline personality disorder	Stage 1b interventions plus case management, educational/vocational intervention/rehabilitation, family psychoeducation and support, specific time-limited psychotherapy, specific and targeted pharmacotherapy (e.g., mood stabilizer)

TABLE 2–2. **A potential clinical-staging model for bipolar disorder and borderline personality disorder** *(continued)*

Clinical stage	Definition	Potential interventions
3a	Recurrence of subthreshold mood or borderline personality disorder symptoms	Stage 2 interventions plus emphasis on maintenance medication and psychosocial strategies for full remission
3b	First threshold relapse of mood disorder or borderline personality disorder	Stage 3a interventions plus relapse-prevention strategies
3c	Multiple relapses of mood disorder or borderline personality disorder	Stage 3b interventions plus combination of mood stabilizers and intensive psychosocial interventions (e.g., dialectical behavior therapy)
4	Persistent, unremitting disorder	Stage 3c interventions plus clozapine and other tertiary therapies, and social participation despite disability

Note.   HYPE=Helping Young People Early.
Source.   Republished with permission of the President and Fellows of Harvard College and Wolters Kluwer Health Inc. from Chanen AM, Berk M, Thompson K: "Integrating Early Intervention for Borderline Personality Disorder and Mood Disorders." *Harvard Review of Psychiatry* 24(5):330–341, 2016. Permission conveyed through Copyright Clearance Center, Inc.

that in a care system without early intervention at mild or developing stages, during which the disease course is more malleable, patients often need to present with suicidality to receive care. This phenomenon leads to a bias of clinicians that all patients with BPD have high acuity and complex clinical profiles. Chanen and colleagues argue that this clinical impression is created by the practice of waiting too long to intervene in problems of BPD.

Chanen's model is divided into four clinical stages. Individuals with increased risk for mood disorders and BPD (Stage 0)—that is, those with family history, childhood adversity, or substance abuse—can be identified before developing symptoms and can benefit from basic mental health literacy to increase their awareness of psychiatric problems, availability of treatments, and general measures to promote mental health (e.g., adequate sleep, avoidance of substances). For individuals with early mild or nonspecific symptoms (Stages 1a), psychoeducation, problem-solving support, and general mental health counseling are indicated for risk reduction. Others have proposed these strategies as early interventions for families as well because psychoeducational groups and more emotionally sensitive behaviors by parents—for example, supportive/validating behavior, autonomy-promoting behavior, and consistent warmth and nurturance of positive affect—have been associated with decreases in BPD symptoms, even in individuals not meeting full BPD criteria (Schuppert et al. 2009; Stepp et al. 2012; Whalen et al. 2014). These interventions constitute a general preventive approach for those at risk of developing any psychiatric problems in youth.

Brief generalist care models are recommended for those with mood or BPD subthreshold symptoms (Stage 1b); enhancement of care is recommended following a first episode of symptoms meeting diagnostic criteria (Stage 2). At this stage, the focus is on case management, educational or vocational rehabilitation, family psychoeducation and support, and specific time-limited psychotherapy and targeted pharmacotherapy. With recurrence of subthreshold symptoms or first threshold relapse (Stages 3a and 3b), Chanen and colleagues' model emphasizes maintenance medication and psychosocial strategies for full remission, as well as relapse-prevention strategies. Specialized treatments such as DBT are reserved for recurrent episodes of symptoms meeting diagnostic criteria (Stage 3c). Persistent and unremitting cases are then targeted with medications such as clozapine, as well as social participation in spite of disability (Stage 4). In these later stages of the disorder, the risks of leaving the disorder untreated outweigh the benefits of reducing burden on highly specialized treatment centers.

Chanen and colleagues built this stepped care system specifically with young people in mind, recognizing that early intervention reduces morbidity and mortality. Early intervention can also prevent developmental arrests in emerging adults, who remain at risk of developing elevated levels of BPD pathology later on if their psychological capacities remain impaired (Cohen et al. 2005; Nakar et al. 2016). Chanen and colleagues recognize that early forms of mood and personality disorders in childhood and adolescence often look similar and cannot be diagnostically clarified until subsequent recurrences define the course (Chanen and Thompson 2015). Generic maneuvers, such as sleep hygiene, avoidance of substance use, and stress management skills, are emphasized at these early stages during which premature diagnostic certainty could lead to therapeutic overkill. Although the model was designed for youth, organizing principles around clinical staging is both pragmatic and relatable to most health professionals.

Chanen and colleagues' clinical staging approach to building steps of care makes good general medical sense. For patients with any serious medical condition, clinicians do not wait until the disease has reached advanced stages in order to treat it. What is most sensible is to intervene earlier, when the problems are more contained, focal, and often less severe. At these earlier stages, intervening with less drastic measures allows patients and their families to make milder adjustments focusing on functional concerns rather than purely on symptom reduction. In addition, the earlier interventions are generic in the sense that most clinical settings can provide them. This model proposes distributing more care earlier to reduce the likelihood of broader effects as psychiatric disorders intensify in their clinical stage and reserving those treatments that are currently considered the "gold standard" to later phases, after the person with BPD has attempted less intensive measures.

Stepped Care Model: Specifying Evidence-Based Care at Different Clinical Stages

In 2016, Choi-Kain and colleagues proposed a model of stepped care that extended Chanen and colleagues' (2016) model, integrating their clinical staging with more explicit guidelines on the use of BPD-specific evidence-based treatments, in their full package forms, as well as individual components such as DBT skills training (Figure 2–1) (Choi-Kain and Gunderson 2019; Choi-Kain et al. 2016). Like Chanen and collaborators' clinical stage model, this stepped care proposal starts with psychoeducation, supportive counseling, and problem solving at preclinical stages (i.e., for those at risk or with subthreshold symptoms of BPD).

	Severity	Definition	Potential interventions
5 Chronic persistent	Unremitting disorder Unresponsive to intervention	Unresponsive to interventions from previous stages, due to severity and complexity, or nonadherence to treatment recommendations	GPM (low frequency, e.g., weekly, monthly, or quarterly) Supportive therapy Case management (e.g., state/public services)
4 Severe	Remitting and relapsing	+ Severe self-harm + Potentially fatal suicide attempts	GPM (+ medication management) PLUS Higher level of care Integration of EBTs OR Change EBT (rarely available)
3 Sustained moderate	Sustained threshold-level symptoms	Unresponsive to basic treatment + Self-harm + Suicidal gestures	GPM (+ medication management) PLUS DBT skills, MBT, or STEPPS group when available
2 Early mild	First episode of threshold BPD	+ Self-harm – Suicidality	GPM Case management DBT skills, MBT, or STEPPS group when available; self-help if relevant
1 Preclinical	Subthreshold	Interpersonal hypersensitivity Rejection sensitivity Emotional dysregulation	Psychoeducation and health literacy Focus on problem solving and supportive counseling addressing interpersonal hypersensitivity and rejection sensitivity

FIGURE 2–1.   Stepped care model.

BPD=borderline personality disorder; DBT=dialectical behavior therapy; EBT=evidence-based treatment; GPM=good psychiatric management; MBT=mentalization-based treatment; STEPPS=Systems Training for Emotional Predictability and Problem Solving.
Source.   Adapted from Choi-Kain et al. 2016. Reprinted from Choi-Kain LW, Gunderson JG (eds): *Applications of Good Psychiatric Management for Borderline Personality Disorder: A Practical Guide.* American Psychiatric Association Publishing, Washington, DC, 2019, Copyright © 2019 American Psychiatric Association Publishing. Used with permission.

However, it employs GPM as the basic approach to care at the first episode of full-criteria BPD, reserving specialist evidence-based treatments for those who relapse or do not improve with GPM.

This system allows generalist mental health care staff to provide *good enough* basic care to all patients, while still providing a place for referrals to specialists whose unique training in more intensive psychotherapies equips them to treat patients for whom generic BPD treatment was not effective. This approach is informed by the DBT dismantling study (Linehan et al. 2015) and by evidence that fully packaged adherent evidence-based psychotherapies for BPD cannot be implemented or maintained realistically in most clinical settings (Bales et al. 2017; Carmel et al. 2014; Iliakis et al. 2019; Landes et al. 2017; Swenson et al. 2002).

Step-ups and step-downs in this system can be determined by clinical staging, patient motivation, treatment responsiveness, and access to BPD-specific care. Many patients will continue to stay in GPM because their motivation to enter something more frequent, intensive, and psychotherapeutically specialized may be limited. Additionally, in most areas globally, DBT skills training and other evidence-based treatments will not be available, in which case GPM or general care will remain the staple, although frequency may increase to once weekly with group therapy, if possible.

This stepped care model recommends *step-downs*, or tapering of intensive treatment resources, in chronic cases where the patient remains unresponsive to intensive and specialized treatment (Stage 5). In clinical practice, the patients who are least responsive to care often rotate through the most specialized and intensive forms of care. In this model, however, less specialized services such as supportive therapy and case management can be used for patients at this stage, reserving the short supply of intensive specialized therapies for patients who have not tried them and might benefit from them. In this last stage, the option would remain open for the patient to revisit intensive treatment if their responsiveness to the care that is provided is improved.

This stepped care system was developed in a context in which specialized options for BPD treatment exist but are often inaccessible. As in the models by Paris (2013) and Chanen and colleagues (2016, the stepped care system advocates for briefer, earlier, and less intensive interventions and steps that advance to specialized intensive psychotherapy only for those who need, want, and can access that level of care. This system is described here as employing GPM as a mainstay only because GPM is the subject of this book, but we believe any tested generalist approach that is informed by, structured around, and focused on BPD would be effective.

Ten-Session Good Psychiatric Management

Ueli Kramer and colleagues (2011, 2017) in Lausanne, Switzerland, developed and studied the effectiveness of a 10-session variant of GPM, which improved BPD symptoms, interpersonal problems, distress, and adaptive emotions (Berthoud et al. 2017). This 10-session variant serves as the gateway to any personality disorders psychotherapy treatment in the Lausanne clinic, which has specialists in a variety of empirically validated psychotherapies. This model does not specify levels of care, but rather employs 10 sessions of GPM for either a full assessment and diagnostic clarification or for a brief treatment. It allows most patients to get a brief introductory dose of treatment that has medium to large effects on symptoms and interpersonal functioning, as well as small effects on functioning in a social role (Kramer et al. 2014). The 10-session variant has also been shown to be effective in reducing BPD symptoms for individuals who have both BPD and a substance use disorder (Penzenstadler et al. 2018). Adding a form of therapeutic relationship that emphasizes individualized case formulations results in further improvements and an increased likelihood of entering structured psychotherapy, with treatment gains sustained over 6 months (Kramer et al. 2011, 2014, 2017; Maillard et al. 2020).

In terms of implementation as part of a stepped care system, 10-session *assessment* is indicated for patients with acute or long-term symptoms that lead to impairments in social functioning, whereas 10-session *therapy* is indicated for patients with acute or crisis symptoms who have enough motivation but do not want longer-term treatment (Table 2–3) (Charbon et al. 2019). The 10-session assessment proposes an adequate treatment as needed, documents the patient's history of abandonment fears and rejection sensitivity, and uses psychoeducation to foster engagement in future treatment and alliance. In contrast, the 10-session therapy aims to avoid chronic patient status, clarify a personally meaningful diagnosis, integrate cognitive and affective aspects of interpersonal hypersensitivity, and help the patient generalize gains to everyday life (Table 2–4). Psychoeducation is used to promote self-help and improved use of care, and the clinician will be the recipient of abandonment fears and rejection sensitivity rather than simply documenting it. For both the assessment and therapy versions of 10-session GPM, exploring relationships may be helpful to prevent dropout and to provide examples for psychoeducation.

TABLE 2–3. Two versions of 10-session good psychiatric management: assessment and therapy

	10-session assessment	10-session therapy
Indications	Patients with acute or long-term symptoms, comorbidities, and maladaptive behaviors leading to social functioning impairment	Patients with acute symptoms or crisis symptoms who have enough psychological motivation and do not want to engage in a long psychiatric treatment
Goals	Propose an adequate treatment as needed	Avoid becoming a chronic psychiatric patient
Abandonment fears and rejection sensitivity	Mostly documented while exploring the patient's history and actual real-life relations	Mostly manifested toward the therapy frame and primary clinician
Work on interpersonal relationships	Exploring relationships in the assessment may be helpful to prevent dropout	Exploring relationships in the therapy may be helpful to prevent dropout
	Exploring real life, work, relations, previous treatments provides examples for psychoeducation about interpersonal hypersensitivity	Exploring relationships in therapy provides examples for psychoeducation about interpersonal hypersensitivity
Use of psychoeducation	Fosters engagement in future treatment and alliance	Provides a canvas for future self-help or to improve use of care

Source. Reprinted from Charbon P, Kramer U, Droz J, Kolly S: "Implementation of Good Psychiatric Management in 10 Sessions," in *Applications of Good Psychiatric Management for Borderline Personality Disorder: A Practical Guide.* Edited by Choi-Kain LW, Gunderson JG. Washington, DC, American Psychiatric Association Publishing, 2019, pp. 233–252. Copyright © 2019 American Psychiatric Association Publishing. Used with permission.

TABLE 2–4.   Goals of 10-session therapy

1. Clarification of medical diagnosis	Comprehend symptoms in medical terms, as well as links between BPD and real-life problems; explain false beliefs about BPD.
2. Meaningful psychiatric diagnosis	Recognize links between borderline personality disorder diagnosis as a medical construct and the patient's real-life problems.
3. Cognitive and affective integration of the diagnosis	Recognize importance of affective and cognitive integration of interpersonal hypersensitivity in patient's interpersonal life, outside and inside the therapy.
4. Emphasize importance of adequate goals outside of therapy (e.g., work and love)	Comprehend and integrate good psychiatric management principles in real life.

Note.   BPD=borderline personality disorder.
Source.   Reprinted from Charbon P, Kramer U, Droz J, Kolly S: "Implementation of Good Psychiatric Management in 10 Sessions," in *Applications of Good Psychiatric Management for Borderline Personality Disorder: A Practical Guide.* Edited by Choi-Kain LW, Gunderson JG. Washington, DC, American Psychiatric Association Publishing, 2019, pp. 233–252. Copyright © 2019 American Psychiatric Association Publishing. Used with permission.

This 10-session introductory therapy variant of GPM offers an introduction to the BPD diagnosis and other co-occurring diagnoses, as well as the contextual life problems the patient has at the time of referral to treatment. For some patients, this model can provide a booster of awareness and support that stabilizes patients well enough, and for others it provides a gateway to a longer-term treatment plan with a specialized psychotherapy selected after an in-depth assessment. This brief 10-session therapy is a step in care that can ensure that all patients get general information and advisement related to BPD as a standard, evolving to further levels of intensity and duration only if needed and desired.

Whole of Service Stepped Care Approach

In Australia, Brin Grenyer and colleagues developed a brief stepped care approach to personality disorders (Grenyer et al. 2018). It involves four weekly outpatient sessions immediately available as a step-down from emergency rooms or inpatient hospitalization. This sensitive period between urgent increased level of care and outpatient care represents a time when the suicide rate is 200 times the global rate (Chung et al. 2017) and up to nine times more likely (Haglund et al. 2019) than it would otherwise be within a given diagnostic category. These four sessions focus on 1) exploring factors that led to the crisis and developing a care plan, 2) working on care plan themes, and 3) exploring carer perceptions and developing a carer plan, with psychotherapy, psychoeducation, risk assessment, support, and referral planning throughout.

A study conducted on this model found reduced demand on hospital services, with shorter stays, fewer emergency visits, and an estimated cost savings of $2,720 per patient per year (Grenyer et al. 2018), an amount that was on par with the cost savings of $2,988 per patient per year that was observed with evidence-based treatments for BPD (Meuldijk et al. 2017). In another article about this trial, Huxley and colleagues (2019) reported that at the conclusion of the intervention in one of the clinics, fewer than 43% of patients needed referrals to psychiatric services, and only 13.6% needed to be stepped up to inpatient care.

Grenyer and colleagues have worked to disseminate this intervention through the Project Air Strategy for Personality Disorders, an Australia-based internationally recognized leader in translational research, advocacy, public health policy, education, and treatment for personality disorders. In their intervention, based on generalist treatment guidelines (Bateman et al. 2015) for personality disorders, they recommend the following: 1) structured approaches to personality disorder symptoms; 2) patient self-efficacy and agency; 3) connection of feelings to events and actions; 4) active, responsive, and validating treaters; and 5) therapist consultation and supervision on cases. There are now over 25 brief intervention clinics for personality disorder in Australia, and more clinics are in development. The spreading implementation of this variant of stepped care shows its accessibility and feasibility as a model of care.

Grenyer and colleagues have developed and implemented this pragmatic brief intermediate step of care, which bridges acute moments of increased risk for patients with BPD to stabilization, so that the patients can be in a state that allows them to engage more effectively in a more elaborate or long-term therapy if desired, required, and available. This step of care is clear, focused, and generalizable to most health care settings to reduce the need for lengthy treatment in inpatient or emergency room care when patients are waiting to be connected with longer-term options. If patients with BPD receive this brief step of care immediately rather than when they are in the right position on a waiting list, they may be better able to choose more care or not while in a clearer state of mind and not merely out of urgency.

Stepped Care: Integrating Dialectical Behavior Therapy and Good Psychiatric Management

In our model that integrates GPM and DBT with stepped care, we propose combining Paris's (2013) model of using primarily brief treatments with a clinical staging model like Chanen and colleagues' (2016) that advocates for early intervention. We recommend brief psychoeducation and/or 10-session GPM as the entry point of treatment at the earliest possible point of intervention, when symptoms are subthreshold or reaching criteria at first episode. The key, as noted in the study by Grenyer and colleagues (2018), is for brief treatment to be readily available rather than be so scarce as to generate waiting lists. Those responding to treatment could either step down to intermittent follow-up or continue for a longer course depending on motivation and availability of care.

Models such as GPM can be flexibly adapted to an infrequent schedule of monthly to yearly visits to provide psychiatric monitoring and primary care to patients with BPD who have remission of symptoms. Patients can start with 10 sessions of GPM or short-term GPM, depending on the resources available to the mental health care system adopting stepped care. This approach would ideally allow the majority of patients to receive standard, effective care, while the minority can receive more elaborate and lengthy treatments, such as the gold standard specialist BPD treatments. Regardless of the model, stepped care systems should incorporate resources to assist patients with BPD in vocational activities.

In an analysis of McMain and collaborators' DBT versus GPM trial, the researchers reported three groups of patients: 1) rapid responders who sustain treatment gains, 2) slow responders who sustain gains, and 3) rapid responders who return to baseline postdischarge (McMain et al. 2018). The third group was distinguished by higher baseline depression, high utilization of health care, and unemployment. McMain and collaborators suggest this third group may need modifications to their treatment targeting these features. Specifically, they argue occupational functioning is an important treatment target to improve outcomes for this group.

At any level of stepped care, GPM's emphasis on building a life outside treatment should be prioritized. When patients with BPD are encouraged to have a life in which they make contact with others and make a valued contribution in their work, they may have adequate opportunities to manage problems of aloneness and poor self-esteem with less drastic symptomatic measures. Having a more fulfilling life would ultimately reduce their need to rely on treatment for structure, activity, and connection with others. The ultimate goals of DBT and GPM converge in stepped care to help patients focus on being more effective by generalizing their skills outside of treatment and building a life that feels worth living; this allows individuals with BPD to be more than patients. Too often, people with BPD become full-time patients because of the way their symptoms interrupt continuous goal-oriented activities and because of the demands of some of the intensive specialized treatments. Because of the short supply and stringent requirements of these specialized treatments, oftentimes patients have no choice but to go to group or appointments that might interfere with fulfilling other responsibilities outside of treatment.

Stepped care models allow for judicious allocation of resource-intensive treatments, to create a multifaceted system and overall more accessible care for patients with BPD. Considering that evidence-based treatment of patients with BPD results in cost savings of around $2,988 per patient per year (Meuldijk et al. 2017), treating BPD more broadly and effectively would yield substantial cost savings and mitigate the unreasonably long waitlists for more intensive psychotherapeutic follow-up. Allocating more care with less intensity, shorter duration, and earlier in a patient's trajectory may lead to the best outcomes for patients, the clinicians who treat them, and the health care system at large. Further research is needed to test these claims, but the preliminary evidence holds promise that clinicians can do less for more and still achieve good enough outcomes.

Key Points

- More easily implementable generalist treatments like GPM and more resource-intensive specialist treatments like DBT have important places in stepped care systems, which provide different intensities of care depending on the patient's clinical severity, the patient's responsiveness and motivation for treatment, and the treatment's availability.

- Various models of stepped care emphasize briefer treatments, less intensive preventive interventions, clinical staging, intermediate step-downs from acute care settings, lower levels of longer-term maintenance, and gateways to more intensive longer-term treatment.

- GPM and DBT can be integrated into a stepped care model by beginning with briefer care such as psychoeducation and/or 10-session GPM as an entry point to treatment as soon as symptoms are detected, followed by a step-down to intermittent follow-up or a step-up to longer-term treatments such as GPM in combination with DBT skills group or comprehensive DBT, depending on what is desired, needed, and available.

References

Bales DL, Verheul R, Hutsebaut J: Barriers and facilitators to the implementation of mentalization-based treatment (MBT) for borderline personality disorder. Personal Ment Health 11(2):118–131, 2017

Bateman AW, Gunderson J, Mulder R: Treatment of personality disorder. Lancet 385(9969):735–743, 2015

Berthoud L, Pascual-Leone A, Caspar F, et al: Leaving distress behind: a randomized controlled study on change in emotional processing in borderline personality disorder. Psychiatry 80(2):139–154, 2017

Brodsky BS, Stanley B: The Dialectical Behavior Therapy Primer: How DBT Can Inform Clinical Practice. Hoboken, NJ, Wiley, 2013

Carmel A, Rose ML, Fruzzetti AE: Barriers and solutions to implementing dialectical behavior therapy in a public behavioral health system. Adm Poly Ment Health Ment Health Serv Res 41:608–614, 2014

Chanen AM, Thompson K: Borderline personality and mood disorders: risk factors, precursors, and early signs in childhood and youth, in Borderline Personality and Mood Disorders: Comorbidity and Controversy. Edited by Choi-Kain LW, Gunderson JG. New York, Springer, 2015, pp 155–174

Chanen AM, Berk M, Thompson K: Integrating early intervention for borderline personality disorder and mood disorders. Harv Rev Psychiatry 24(5):330–341, 2016

Charbon P, Kramer U, Droz J, Kolly S: Implementation of good psychiatric management in 10 sessions, in Applications of Good Psychiatric Management for Borderline Personality Disorder: A Practical Guide. Edited by Choi-Kain LW, Gunderson JG. Washington, DC, American Psychiatric Association Publishing, 2019, pp 233–252

Choi-Kain LW, Gunderson JG (eds): Applications of Good Psychiatric Management for Borderline Personality Disorder: A Practical Guide. Washington, DC, American Psychiatric Association Publishing, 2019

Choi-Kain LW, Albert EB, Gunderson JG: Evidence-based treatments for borderline personality disorder: implementation, integration, and stepped care. Harv Rev Psychiatry 24(5):342–356, 2016

Choi-Kain LW, Finch EF, Masland SR, et al: What works in the treatment of borderline personality disorder. Curr Behav Neurosci Rep 4(1):21–30, 2017a

Choi-Kain LW, Glasserman EI, Finch EF: Borderline personality disorder: treatment resistance reconsidered. Psychiatric Times 34(11), 2017b

Chung DT, Ryan CJ, Hadzi-Pavlovic D, et al: Suicide rates after discharge from psychiatric facilities: a systematic review and meta-analysis. JAMA Psychiatry 74(7):694–702, 2017

Cohen P, Crawford TN, Johnson JG, Kasen S: The children in the community study of developmental course of personality disorder. J Pers Disord 19(5):466–486, 2005

Cristea IA, Gentili C, Cotet CD, et al: Efficacy of psychotherapies for borderline personality disorder: a systematic review and meta-analysis. JAMA Psychiatry 74(4):319–328, 2017

Grenyer BFS, Lewis KL, Fanaian M, et al: Treatment of personality disorder using a whole of service stepped care approach: a cluster randomized controlled trial. PLoS One 13(11):e0206472, 2018

Gunderson JG, Links PS: Borderline Personality Disorder: A Clinical Guide, 2nd Edition. Washington, DC, American Psychiatric Publishing, 2008

Gunderson JG, Links PS: Handbook of Good Psychiatric Management for Borderline Personality Disorder. Washington, DC, American Psychiatric Publishing, 2014

Haglund A, Lysell H, Larsson H, et al: Suicide immediately after discharge from psychiatric inpatient care: a cohort study of nearly 2.9 million discharges. J Clin Psychiatry 80(2):27–32, 2019

Huxley E, Lewis KL, Coates AD, et al: Evaluation of a brief intervention within a stepped care whole of service model for personality disorder. BMC Psychiatry 19(1):341, 2019

Iliakis EA, Sonley AKI, Ilagan GS, et al: Treatment of borderline personality disorder: Is supply adequate to meet public health needs? Psychiatr Serv 70(9):772–781, 2019

Knight RP: Management and psychotherapy of the borderline schizophrenic patient. Bull Menninger Clin 17(4):139–150, 1953

Kramer U, Berger T, Kolly S, et al: Effects of motive-oriented therapeutic relationship in early phase treatment of borderline personality disorder: a pilot study of a randomized trial. J Nerv Ment Dis 199(4):244–250, 2011

Kramer U, Kolly S, Berthoud L, et al: Effects of motive-oriented therapeutic relationship in a ten-session general psychiatric treatment of borderline personality disorder: a randomized controlled trial. Psychother Psychosom 83(3):176–186, 2014

Kramer U, Stulz N, Berthoud L, et al: The shorter the better? A follow-up analysis of 10-session psychiatric treatment including the motive-oriented psychotherapeutic relationship for borderline personality disorder. Psychother Res 27(3):362–370, 2017

Landes SJ, Rodriguez AL, Smith BN, et al: Barriers, facilitators, and benefits of implementation of dialectical behavior therapy in routine care: results from a national program evaluation survey in the Veterans Health Administration. Transl Behav Med 7:832–844, 2017

Laporte L, Paris J, Bergevin T, et al: Clinical outcomes of a stepped care program for borderline personality disorder. Personal Ment Health 12(3):252–264, 2018

Linehan MM, Korslund KE, Harned MS, et al: Dialectical behavior therapy for high suicide risk in individuals with borderline personality disorder: a randomized clinical trial and component analysis. JAMA Psychiatry 72(5):475–482, 2015

Maillard P, Dimaggio G, Berthoud L, et al: Metacognitive improvement and symptom change in a 3-month treatment for borderline personality disorder. Psychol Psychother 93(2):309–235, 2020

McMain SF, Fitzpatrick S, Boritz T, et al: Outcome trajectories and prognostic factors for suicide and self-harm behaviors in patients with borderline personality disorder following one year of outpatient psychotherapy. J Pers Disord 32(4):497–512, 2018

Meuldijk D, McCarthy A, Bourke ME, et al: The value of psychological treatment for borderline personality disorder: systematic review and cost offset analysis of economic evaluations. PLoS One 12(3):e0171592, 2017

Nakar O, Brunner R, Schilling O, et al: Developmental trajectories of self-injurious behavior, suicidal behavior and substance misuse and their association with adolescent borderline personality pathology. J Affect Disord 197:231–238, 2016

Neacsiu AD, Rizvi SL, Linehan MM: Dialectical behavior therapy skills use as a mediator and outcome of treatment for borderline personality disorder. Behav Res Ther 48(9):632–639, 2010

Paris J: Stepped care: an alternative to routine extended treatment for patients with borderline personality disorder. Psychiatr Serv 64(10):1035–1037, 2013

Paris J: Stepped Care for Borderline Personality Disorder: Making Treatment Brief, Effective, and Accessible. Cambridge, MA, Academic Press, 2017

Penzenstadler L, Kolly S, Rothen S, et al: Effects of substance use disorder on treatment process and outcome in a ten-session psychiatric treatment for borderline personality disorder. Subst Abuse Treat Prev Policy 13(1):10, 2018

Quaytman M, Sharfstein SS: Treatment for severe borderline personality disorder in 1987 and 1997. Am J Psychiatry 154(8):1139–1144, 1997

Schuppert HM, Giesen-Bloo J, van Gemert TG, et al: Effectiveness of an emotion regulation group training for adolescents: a randomized controlled pilot study. Clin Psychol Psychother 16(6):467–478, 2009

Stepp SD, Whalen DJ, Pilkonis PA, et al: Children of mothers with borderline personality disorder: identifying parenting behaviors as potential targets for intervention. Personal Disord 3(1):76–91, 2012

Stoffers JM, Völlm BA, Rücker G, et al: Psychological therapies for people with borderline personality disorder. Cochrane Database Syst Rev (8):CD005652, 2012

Swenson CR, Torrey WC, Koerner K: Implementing dialectical behavior therapy. Psychiatr Serv 53:171–178, 2002

Whalen DJ, Scott LN, Jakubowski KP, et al: Affective behavior during mother–daughter conflict and borderline personality disorder severity across adolescence. Personal Disord 5(1):88–96, 2014

3

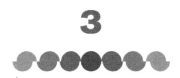

Basics of Good Psychiatric Management and Dialectical Behavior Therapy Treatment

Deanna Mercer, M.D., FRCPC

Anne K.I. Sonley, J.D., M.D., FRCPC

Lois W. Choi-Kain, M.D., M.Ed.

In this chapter we outline basic strategies to start and guide treatment when working with someone with borderline personality disorder. The first section, on clinician stance, includes clarifications of commonly held beliefs about borderline personality disorder (BPD) that can interfere with clinician empathy, strategies to build an effective alliance, and guidance around the therapeutic use of self-disclosure and irreverence. The second section covers three tasks that are important when starting treatment, including providing psychoeducation about the diagnosis of BPD, discussing the frequency and length of treatment with the patient, and helping the patient identify "life worth living" goals. The final section provides a framework for ongoing treatment, including a suggested structure, content, and approach within sessions.

Clinician Stance

Given that interpersonal instability and emotional intensity are symptoms of BPD, clinicians can sometimes have difficulty maintaining an alliance with patients with BPD. When people grow up with heightened emotional and social sensitivities and then encounter repeated invalidating and traumatic experiences, they naturally often adapt by becoming less trusting and less open to others. The resulting vigilance, reactivity, and difficulties with social learning that people with BPD develop are not surprising and can lead clinicians to experience these individuals as "difficult patients." Understandably, it can be more difficult for a clinician to provide treatment when a patient's trust and openness is limited. Dialectical behavior therapy (DBT) and good psychiatric management (GPM) suggest specific strategies to enhance clinician empathy, as well as strategies to build a good working alliance with patients who may tend not to be naturally trusting and open. Maintaining an empathetic stance is useful regardless of whether a clinician is seeing a patient for one session, longer-term therapy, or anything in between.

Empathy and Addressing Stigma

GPM and DBT both provide a framework for the clinician to connect with patients empathically and serve to reduce clinician stigma toward patients with BPD. John Gunderson began his career with the important observation that patients with BPD were poorly understood and received treatments that were not suited to them, which explained why they were not responding to treatment as expected. Gunderson noted that there are commonly held "myths" that contribute to the significant stigma regarding BPD and that interfere with effective treatment (Gunderson 1984; Gunderson and Links 2014) (Table 3–1). Several myths about BPD (myths 1–3 listed in Table 3–1) have fueled a lack of recognition that the problems that arise in the therapeutic alliance are symptoms of the disorder for which the patient seeks treatment. For example, myth 1—that people with BPD angrily attack their treaters—can instead be recast in terms of the excessive anger and fearfulness of others that are symptoms of BPD. When these personality characteristics are not named as central symptoms to be managed, both the patient and clinician are prone to overly personalize interpersonal conflicts that occur. This is even more harmful to the patient if the clinician does not share the BPD diagnosis with the patient who feels bad or evil rather than ill and in need of help.

By taking a medicalized framework of understanding BPD as the central problem, clinicians are able to be more prepared and focused on teaching their patients what they need to learn so they can better manage their interpersonal vulnerabilities and get what they need from relationships. Clarification of these myths therefore can shift wariness toward the patient with BPD to a more empathic position. The myth that people with BPD rarely get better (myth 2) can breed hopelessness

TABLE 3–1.   Common myths about borderline personality disorder (BPD)

Myth	GPM Clarification
1. People with BPD angrily attack their treaters.	Excessive anger and fearfulness of treaters are symptoms of the disorder.
2. People with BPD rarely get better.	10% remit within 6 months, 25% by 1 year, and 50% by 2 years. Relapses are unusual.
3. People with BPD get better only if given intensive treatment by experts.	Such treatment is needed only by a subsample.
4. People with BPD resist treatment.	Most seek relief from their pain, and seek treatment following psychoeducation.
5. Recurrent risk of suicide burdens treaters with serious liability risks.	Excessive burden or fears of litigation are symptoms of poorly structured treatments.
6. Recurrent crises require treaters to be available 24/7.	Such a requirement is rare and may mean a different level of care is needed.
7. BPD traits are "character flaws" or moral deficits.	Although individuals with BPD often see themselves as being "bad" or "evil," BPD traits are rooted in genetics and learned behaviors.

Note.   GPM=good psychiatric management.
Source.   Adapted from Gunderson and Links 2014.

but can be counteracted with psychoeducation reviewing research showing that the vast majority of patients remit from symptoms over time. GPM also was designed to counteract myths that intensive treatment by experts and around-the-clock clinician availability are necessary for effective treatment (myths 3 and 6). DBT, an intensive treatment that provides around-the-clock skills coaching in its complete form, is not the only treatment that works for BPD, and generalist approaches are now recognized as good enough (see Chapter 2, "Integration of Good Psychiatric Management and Dialectical Behavior Therapy With Stepped Care for Borderline Personality Disorder"). Dispelling these commonly held misunderstandings regarding BPD using up-to-date medical knowledge can restore the faith of both clinicians and patients in the work they can do together.

In DBT, clinicians and patients are given a set of assumptions that they agree to adopt (Table 3–2). These assumptions (e.g., assumption 2, that people with BPD want to improve) have the effect of reducing clinicians' sense of futility or negative feelings toward patients and can also reduce patients' negative judgments of themselves. In DBT, it is recommended that a clinician review the DBT assumptions with patients at the beginning of treatment. These assumptions become the foundation of how the patient and clinician understand their work together. They clearly lay out roles and goals that are equally applicable to both clinician and patient. They instruct the clinician and patient to understand what causes emotions and behaviors to change, rather than judging or blaming. They also pose the expectation that new behavior must be learned in all relevant contexts, which frames an expectation that what is learned in treatment is to be used outside of treatment.

Alliance Building

At the beginning of treatment, the alliance between patient and clinician is often the only reason a patient stays in treatment. It is generally not until treatment progresses, and a patient has experienced improvement in life outside of treatment, that the patient has confidence in the treatment. GPM and DBT include strategies to help build a strong therapeutic alliance in order to engage a patient in treatment. Both treatments involve the following:

- Psychoeducation: Psychoeducation about the disorder reduces shame and instills hope that treatment will be effective.
- Active stance and direct communication: An active, engaged, and conversational stance is encouraged. Direct and open communication with the patient about what the clinician is thinking and experiencing in session is likely to improve trust and openness to new learning. Unclear communication, such as extended periods of silence, is often extremely anxiety provoking and aversive.
- Validation: Expressing genuine curiosity about and understanding of the patient's experience is called *validation*. Validating patients'

TABLE 3–2.   Dialectical behavior therapy (DBT) assumptions

1. People with BPD are doing the best that they can.

2. People with BPD want to improve.

3. People with BPD need to do better, try harder, and be more motivated to change.

4. People with BPD may not have caused all of their own problems, but they have to solve them anyway.

5. The lives of suicidal individuals with BPD are unbearable as they are currently being lived.

6. New behavior has to be learned in all relevant contexts.

7. All behaviors (actions, thoughts, emotions) are caused.

8. Figuring out and changing the cause of behavior is a more effective way to change than judging and blaming.

9. Clients cannot fail in therapy.

10. Clinicians treating clients with BPD need support.

Note.   BPD=borderline personality disorder.
Source.   Adapted with permission of Guilford Publications Inc. from Linehan MM: "Overview of Treatment: Targets, Strategies, and Assumptions in a Nutshell," in *Cognitive-Behavioral Treatment of Borderline Personality Disorder*. New York, Guilford, 1993, pp. 106–108. Permission conveyed through Copyright Clearance Center, Inc.

distress helps to reduce their distress and helps patients to feel understood by the clinician, strengthening the therapeutic alliance. (Validation is discussed more fully in Chapter 5, "Dialectical Behavior Therapy Tool Kit.")

- Addressing situational stressors and distress: Clinicians are encouraged to inquire about and address current problems that patients are experiencing in day-to-day living. Effectiveness and mastery in dealing with "here-and-now" problems and the subsequent reduction in subjective distress strengthen the therapeutic alliance.

- Clinician consistency and confidence: The structure and strategies of the treatments have been demonstrated to be effective for helping patients to reduce distress, cope with overwhelming emotions, and build a life worth living. Having structure increases a clinician's ability to respond consistently to patients. A clinician's confidence in the effectiveness of the interventions engages the patient, who in the past may have encountered clinicians who were uncertain whether any treatment could be effective. At the same time, clinician confidence needs to be tempered with the realization that no treatment is universally effective.

- Clinician availability: In general, patients with BPD find therapy difficult. Usually, they want to feel close to their clinician, but at the same time, they are afraid of this experience. They are hopeful that therapy will change them but are simultaneously very fearful of change. They want to be able to tolerate distress yet often have no confidence that they will be able to get through extreme distress on their own. The offer of intersession clinician support reduces anxiety and avoidance of therapy. This is true even though the majority of patients never contact the clinician outside of regular appointments (Gunderson and Links 2014).

Use of Self-Disclosure and Irreverence

GPM and DBT encourage clinician self-disclosure within limits. Self-disclosure is encouraged when it is in the interest of the patient and is felt to be useful to the treatment. In DBT, there are two types of self-disclosure: self-involving and personal (Linehan 1993).

In a *self-involving disclosure*, the clinician shares immediate personal reactions to patient behavior. For example, a clinician might disclose, "When you scream at me like that, I feel scared and it makes it hard for me to concentrate on helping you," or "It's hard for me when you repeatedly tell me that I'm not helping you. It's leaving me feeling demotivated." Through self-involving self-disclosure, the clinician provides the patient with an understanding of what the clinician is thinking or feeling, as well as important feedback about the effect of the patient's behaviors on others. This type of disclosure also models accurate and direct communication.

Personal self-disclosure involves sharing past experiences the clinician has had to model either normative responses or ways to deal with problems. For example, when teaching a patient a skill, a clinician might describe a situation in which that skill was used and found to be useful.

Self-disclosure of personal information is limited to information the clinician is comfortable sharing. When uncomfortable with providing the information requested, the clinician is not obliged to share this information. However, it is important that the clinician not imply that the patient's desire for more disclosure is pathological. Although self-disclosure can be helpful, the clinician should avoid burdening a patient with the clinician's problems. It is also important for the clinician not to invalidate the patient by making an assumption about the similarities between the clinician's and the patient's difficulties.

In GPM, the relationship between clinician and patient is both professional and real. Self-involving self-disclosure is used as a mode of providing candid and needed feedback about how the patient's actions affect others, including the clinician. One important area of modeling in GPM involves self-disclosure around making mistakes. Clinicians are advised to admit to mistakes when they happen to communicate that everyone makes mistakes at times, and this means neither that the clinician is bad nor that he or she wanted to be harmful.

Speaking to patients in a matter-of-fact way and using irreverence at times is encouraged in both DBT and GPM. In DBT, *irreverence* refers to providing an offbeat, spontaneous, humorous, or unexpected response to provoke a shift in a patient's thinking or mood (Linehan 1993). Irreverence can throw patients "off balance" a little bit so they are in less of a fixed position and more open to what a clinician is saying. For example, an irreverent response to a patient saying "I'm going to kill myself!" might be "The problem with suicide, of course, is that if you are dead, you won't have me to help you" or "I thought you agreed not to drop out of therapy." Moments of irreverence are generally brief because the predominant clinician stance is to be warm, responsive, engaged, genuine, friendly, and affectionate. Also, the irreverent statement needs to come from a place of genuine compassion and warmth within the clinician, not from annoyance or malice.

Getting Started in Treatment

Making the Diagnosis

One of the most impactful things a clinician can do is to discuss the diagnosis of BPD collaboratively with a patient. Given the stigma associated with BPD within the health care system, it may seem counterintuitive to disclose this diagnosis. However, in our experience, this discussion is usually well received by patients. Research demonstrates that making the diagnosis and providing psychoeducation can result in a reduction in symptoms (Zanarini and Frankenburg 2008; Zanarini et al. 2018). One way to approach the discussion of the diagnosis is to give the patient a copy of the BPD criteria from DSM-5 (American Psychiatric Association 2013) and discuss which criteria the patient feels are a fit for them. Follow this by providing information about etiology, treatment, and prognosis. Note that validating the patient's experience and eliciting personal examples are also very helpful.

The following is a psychoeducation example:

- Review the criteria: "Based on what you have told me so far, I am wondering if your symptoms could be explained by borderline personality disorder. It is a common problem that many people face and can overcome. It can explain, for instance, why you have not had the improvements you were hoping for from the medication treatments or therapies for your anxiety disorder. Here are the criteria for this condition [give patient a printout of the DSM-5 BPD criteria]. Do you think any of these describe you?"

- Elicit curiosity about the etiology of the diagnosis: "Would you like to hear a bit about how this condition develops?"

- Explain the influence of biology: "If you go into a fifth-grade classroom and measure the heights of all the kids, you generally find that some are really tall, some are really short, and most are somewhere in the middle. Most things in nature occur in this pattern. The same goes for emotional intensity: some people are born more emotionally intense, others are born not very emotionally intense, and most people are somewhere in the middle. People with BPD generally tend to experience emotions more intensely than other people do, they are more sensitive to their environment, and their emotions tend to last longer. How would you describe yourself in terms of emotional intensity?"

- Explain the influence of the environment: "Emotional intensity isn't a problem in itself, and many emotionally intense people do not develop BPD. However, for some, their intensity and the environment in which they grow up can be a poor fit. For example, a well-meaning parent might not understand why one of their children is emotionally fine while watching a sad movie, but the other child is still crying 30 minutes after the movie ends. Eventually, a parent might say, 'That's enough, stop crying, it isn't that sad.' For a child, repeated experiences of people not understanding their emotional intensity and sensitivity can lead them to be confused and question their emotional experiences. The term *invalidation* is used to describe this experience of being misunderstood. Traumatic experiences, such as childhood abuse, are considered extreme forms of invalidation. Do you recall experiencing invalidation growing up?"

- Discuss how maladaptive behavior is used to cope: "Having their emotional experience misunderstood often leads people to try and dampen their emotional experience. Many of the symptoms of BPD, such as self-harm, substance use, and binge eating, are thought to be coping mechanisms to dampen emotions. These behaviors tend to work to dampen emotions in the short run, but they sometimes have negative consequences in the long run. How does that fit for you?"

- Examine level of interpersonal sensitivity: "For most people, interpersonal rejection, or worry about being rejected, is distressing. It is not uncommon for people with BPD to become angry or depressed in response to interpersonal rejection. Have you ever noticed that?"

- Discuss treatment and prognosis: "The first step in improving BPD involves making connections between events in the environment, emotions, and behaviors, and noticing patterns that are typical for you. The next step is to help you find alternative, less harmful coping mechanisms. It is also important to know that, as with most other medical conditions, the development of BPD involves both genetic factors and environmental factors. The good news is that most people with BPD get better with time, even without treatment. Do you have any questions?"

Discussing Treatment Frequency and Duration

During the first session with a patient, the clinician should discuss treatment frequency (e.g., weekly, biweekly, monthly) and treatment duration. Treatment may be time limited (e.g., 1 year) or open-ended and based on progress. Standard DBT usually involves four orientation/commitment sessions in which the clinician and patient discuss treatment goals. Treatment does not start until a strong commitment is obtained from the patient with regard to the goals and the treatment. In GPM, it usually takes 1 or 2 sessions to provide the patient with psychoeducation about BPD and obtain commitment to treatment.

In most treatment settings, those patients with more severe BPD receive more treatment. This increase in treatment can be problematic because it can reinforce illness behavior rather than reinforce progress and change. Although GPM and DBT have different approaches to this issue, both therapies agree that continuation of treatment should be dependent on progress in treatment.

In GPM, at the start of treatment, the clinician communicates that treatment will continue only as long as it is shown to be helpful. The frequency of sessions should be tailored based on the patient's progress.

For example, at the beginning of treatment, weekly or even twice-weekly appointments may be useful, as long as the patient is clearly working on the goals and making attempts to use the treatment. If the treatment does not appear to be helpful, then actually reducing the frequency of sessions or ending treatment altogether might be indicated.

In standard DBT, the treatment contract is for 1 year, and the only formal termination rule is that a patient who misses 4 scheduled sessions in a row is out of treatment.

When a patient is not improving, both GPM and DBT recommend reevaluating the treatment. GPM describes clear benchmarks for improvement, as discussed in Chapter 6, "Good Psychiatric Management Tool Kit." Failure to meet those benchmarks prompts the clinician to discuss with the patient the effectiveness of the treatment and to explore what needs to be done to improve treatment. This discussion is an opportunity to refocus and jointly evaluate why they are not seeing progress. If a patient's suicidality is not decreasing, the GPM clinician will openly question whether the treatment is useful. Clinicians should look for ways in which they may be unintentionally reinforcing suicide, such as by giving more attention during crises or by provoking suicidal behaviors through being too nurturing or too distant. Other common indications that the helpfulness of treatment needs to be reevaluated include a patient's persistent intoxication, nonattendance, nonpayment, or refusal to adopt a reasonable safety plan. Treatment will be suspended only after the clinician has concluded that the patient's behaviors are incompatible with the patient's safety or are incompatible with the clinician's ability to be helpful. Upon termination of treatment, the clinician might suggest a referral to a more intensive BPD-specific therapy.

In DBT lack of progress in treatment is handled slightly differently. Behaviors that interfere with the patient getting the most out of the treatment are explored nonjudgmentally, and attempts are made to problem-solve ways to reduce treatment interfering behavior. As a last resort, a DBT clinician may consider placing the patient on a "vacation." During a vacation the patient is "out of treatment" for a specified period of time or until a certain change is made. What the client needs to do to avoid going on vacation or to return from vacation should be behaviorally specific and clear to the patient. During the vacation the clinician is encouraged to contact the patient periodically to let the patient know that they want to keep working with them and hope the patient will do what is needed to return from vacation. Unilateral termination is discouraged in DBT, though a patient may be on vacation until the end of the treatment period (usually 1 year in DBT), after which the patient could re-apply for treatment. In extreme circumstances, if a therapist did decide to terminate treatment, it would be important to emphasize to the patient that the termination indicates a failure of the treatment and not the failure of the patient themselves.

For each practitioner, choosing whether to approach treatment duration and frequency in a flexible way, with a 1-year contract, or with some combination of the two will likely depend on the resources available and the clinical setting in which the treatment occurs. The main principle remains that treatment frequency and duration should be discussed with the patient at the outset of treatment, and then treatment should continue only if it is found to be helpful. In other words, the frequency of treatment is not increased when symptoms are not reduced, and more treatment is applied only if it is working. If treatment is not helping, the patient and clinician need to reevaluate it in a collaborative way.

Identifying Patient Goals

GPM and DBT both emphasize the need to identify a patient's goals at the beginning of treatment. Patients need to be active participants in their treatment, and collaboratively identifying goals is therefore of utmost importance. Working toward achieving patient-identified goals also helps to strengthen the therapeutic alliance.

Both GPM and DBT place a strong focus on the patient's life outside of the treatment and suggest that the overall goal of treatment is to "build a life worth living." What constitutes a life worth living will be different for each individual, and goals, such as reducing self-harm behaviors and attending treatment, are useful in order to meet the primary goal of a better life.

GPM provides suggestions for a life worth living, highlighting the importance of participation in work and building a supportive social network before looking for an intimate relationship. Work is seen as providing structure and is an important source of self-esteem that depends on the patient's activity and contribution rather than on someone else's responsiveness to the patient. A supportive social network provides patients with a sense of security and value. Together, work and social supports help patients with BPD weather the interpersonal stresses of an intimate relationship, which is often the most significant source of their distress.

In GPM, clinicians and patients also develop short-term goals, such as managing or leaving stressful situations, developing the ability to call for support, reducing substance use and self-harm, and improving sleep, which enable the patient to meet the long-term goal of building a life worth living.

In DBT, patients are encouraged to identify their values and goals with respect to what constitutes a life worth living. Sometimes it can be helpful to provide patients with a list of common values and to ask them to rank-order the values in terms of their importance (see Appendix A for a list of common values). Once values are identified, patients are encouraged to set goals that are in line with their values and then to brainstorm smaller action steps to work toward the goals. Values and goals differ in that one's *values* exist in the here and now, whereas *goals* describe what one would like in the future. Action steps are useful because they can be a way to break down goals into smaller steps that are behaviorally specific, measurable, and feasible. For example, a person's value might be "attending to relationships." A goal in line with this value would be "speaking to my parents more often." An action step toward this goal would be "call my parents this Sunday at 7 P.M."

It can be useful for the clinician and patient to identify how goals of 1) decreasing suicidal and life-threatening behaviors, 2) decreasing behaviors that interfere with benefiting from treatment, and 3) decreasing behaviors that interfere with quality of life are related to the patient's values and to identify action steps for working toward these goals.

Although the goal of enhancing a patient's life may seem obvious to clinicians, it is not always so obvious to patients who have often given up hope of improving their lives and are focused on symptom relief. Both GPM and DBT address symptoms and distress, while simultaneously communicating to patients that lasting relief is dependent on improving their lives. Both treatments acknowledge that patients often struggle with setting goals, and clinicians are encouraged to help patients with this task.

Developing a Treatment Contract

All effective BPD treatments need to have a clear treatment framework. It is important to outline from the outset what the clinician can expect of the patient and what the patient can expect from the clinician. These expectations can be discussed verbally or written out. The purpose of this framework is not to create rigidity or inflexibility. It is likely that both the clinician and the patient will step outside of the framework at times. That being said, the framework provides a means to anticipate common difficulties that the clinician and patient might encounter as well as to provide a way to flag and discuss any deviations from the framework.

In addition to providing information regarding frequency and duration of treatment, the clinician needs to be clear from the outset of treatment regarding expectations around the following:

- Commitment to treatment
- Frequency and duration of treatment
- Agreements regarding substance use, self-harm, suicidal behavior, and disordered eating behavior
- Clinician contact with other providers
- Clinician contact with family or other social supports
- Clinician availability outside of office hours (if any)
- Payments
- Missed sessions or lateness
- Requirements for engagement in work, studies, or volunteer commitments
- Plan in case of worsening suicidal ideation

An example of a written treatment contract appears in Appendix B.

Treatment

Session Structure

Having a clear structure is useful when treating BPD because structure can increase the confidence of the clinician and can be containing for the patient. Both GPM and DBT use approaches to individual sessions that create a sense of consistency and predictability for both clinician and patient.

The structure of individual GPM sessions is flexible and can cover a range of topics. GPM sessions typically involve checking on how the patient has been doing since the last appointment and reviewing symptoms that the clinician and patient have agreed are important to work on. Any suicidal behavior, self-harm, or other impulsive behaviors should be addressed. The patient is always encouraged to link events of the week, in particular interpersonal events, to emotions and behaviors, and the clinician aims to help the patient develop a coherent narrative of his or her life: "making sense of yourself and your life" (see Chapter 6, "Good Psychiatric Management Tool Kit").

Individual DBT sessions are more structured. A session opens with reviewing the patient's diary card from the previous week. The patient uses the diary card to record daily target behaviors and urges (e.g., self-harm, substance use), emotions, and skills used over the week (diary cards are described in further detail in Chapter 5, "Dialectical Behavior Therapy Tool Kit"). The patient and clinician then co-create the agenda for the session, with priority given to *target behaviors*. The session finishes with a summary of the session, assigning homework, troubleshooting what might get in the way of doing the homework, and finally highlighting any patient success from the week and in the treatment session.

Making Connections Between Emotions and Behaviors

In DBT and GPM, clinicians assist patients in making connections between current life events and their emotional, cognitive, and behavioral responses. A fundamental assumption in DBT is that all behavior is caused (see Table 3–2, earlier in this chapter, for list of DBT assumptions). It follows that to change a behavior, one must explore what causes the behavior. For example, if a patient wants to eliminate self-harm, it is important to explore examples of times when self-harm has occurred to find out what motivates or leads up to the self-harm (precipitant) and what consequences come afterward and may maintain it (reinforcers). A *chain analysis* is a systematic way of identifying events, emotions, and thoughts that lead to an unwanted behavior and then to consequences, both positive (and reinforcing) and negative, that follow the behavior (Figure 3–1). Once these links are made, it is easier to problem solve around how the different links can be modified in the future to avoid the problem behavior.

A chain analysis can be done verbally, but it also can be useful to have a patient record a chain analysis on a whiteboard or worksheet. The clinician works collaboratively with the patient, helping the patient become curious about and reflect on his or her behavior. The clinician encourages the patient to bring the situation to life emotionally and helps the patient identify the relevant factors and patterns of behavior. It is important that the patient understand the function or essence of the problematic behavior. For example, as a patient and clinician are getting to know each other, more lengthy chain analyses might be appropriate to try to observe common patterns in the patient's chains. Also, if a patient has a persistent behavior that is not changing, it may be that certain factors are being overlooked, and this behavior may warrant more attention and precise analysis.

As a patient becomes more aware of their own behavior patterns, or if the function of the behavior is clear, chain analyses can be conducted more briefly. The following is an example:

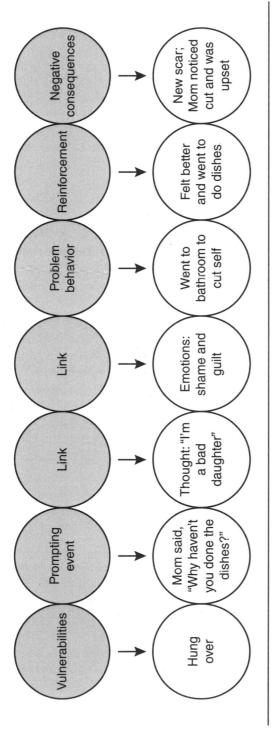

FIGURE 3–1. Sample chain analysis.

Clinician: "What happened yesterday?"
Patient: "I was fired from my job and was feeling a lot of shame. When I walked home, I saw my old dealer on my doorstep. I had a strong urge to use and numb out, so I did."

With time, patients are also encouraged to complete a chain analysis on their own before a session and then review it in session.

It is important to recognize that many patients experience conducting a chain analysis as aversive because it can stimulate recollections of behaviors that may be associated with painful emotions, such as shame. The clinician can be helpful by validating how difficult doing a chain analysis can be and pointing out that to change behavior, the patient must first understand the function or essence of the behavior.

Like DBT, GPM also encourages chain analysis, with the main difference being that in GPM there is more focus on identifying possible interpersonal events that prompt problem behaviors. Both approaches to chain analysis enable the patient to construct an understandable narrative surrounding problematic behaviors.

Active Case Management Approach

Case Management

In both GPM and DBT, clinicians take on a *case management* role with their patients. To clarify what is meant by case management, we can contrast GPM and DBT with other forms of treatment. For example, in classic psychodynamic psychotherapy, what happens in treatment is presumed to reflect what has happened in the patient's early relationships, a situation that is called *transference*. The patient's behaviors in current relationships are interpreted through the lens of the patient's childhood relationships. Much of the focus of a session is on what is happening in the transference relationship between the patient and the clinician.

In contrast to psychodynamic psychotherapy, GPM and DBT focus more on what is happening in the here-and-now in the patient's life outside of treatment. Acting much like a case manager, the clinician pays attention to the patient's activities of daily living, things that are happening with respect to work and family initiatives, budget, and self-care. In GPM, the clinician uses the relationship with the patient as a source of information about what might be happening in relationships outside the treatment. However, psychodynamic strategies of interpretation and confrontation are used rarely, if at all. The clinician works to develop a strong therapeutic alliance with the patient through active attempts to understand and validate the patient's experience. The clinician also makes efforts to help the patient improve his or her life and the quality of relationships outside of treatment.

DBT also focuses on the patient's life outside of treatment and tends toward behavioral formulation over psychodynamic formulation, although childhood experiences can inform this behavioral formulation in terms of the patient's learning history. Clinicians work with patients on problem solving and coaching around goals related to school or work, self-care, and interpersonal relationships.

Active Clinician, Active Patient

The active approach, common to all effective treatments for BPD, differs from therapeutic approaches in which there are long periods during which the patient speaks and the clinician listens, such as in the traditional practice of psychoanalysis. Open-ended, unstructured, psychoanalytic treatments have been found to be ineffective and even harmful to patients with BPD (Gunderson 1984; Gunderson et al. 1989; Waldinger and Gunderson 1984). Extended periods of silence on the part of the clinician are likely to be experienced by the patient as aversive and allow for misinterpretations of what the clinician is feeling or thinking. Many patients with BPD have had invalidating and traumatic experiences in childhood and therefore struggle with trusting others. Long periods of silence tend to induce overwhelming and unhelpful anxiety in the patient with BPD. To increase trust, the clinician is encouraged to use a direct, active, and conversational approach, as well as to openly share the treatment plan and their own thoughts and feelings.

It is also important that patients take an active role in treatment to allow for meaningful change to occur. As mentioned previously, the clinician and patient collaborate in developing goals for the treatment. Patients are also encouraged to be active in session by adding what they would like to discuss in session to the agenda, observing problems they encounter between sessions, completing homework, and collaborating in the problem-solving process with the clinician in session.

Attending Groups

GPM is a generalist treatment designed to be offered by a single clinician; however, GPM strongly encourages patients to be involved in group therapy. Involvement of a patient in a DBT "skills only" group while continuing to see a primary GPM clinician is compatible with the GPM model. GPM proposes that virtually any group that is structured and has an active leader—including support groups, 12-step or recovery groups, interpersonal groups, or mentalization-based treatment groups—can be helpful for people with BPD.

A GPM clinician who is providing individual treatment to a patient who is also in a DBT skills group may find it helpful to know about the structure, content, and expectations of a DBT skills group. DBT skills groups usually have two group leaders and 8–12 patients in a group. The groups generally run for around 2 hours. The first half of a session consists of a mindfulness exercise, followed by review of homework. In the second half, a new skill is taught. Discussing the details of self-injurious behavior, substance use, and other impulsive behaviors is actively discouraged in skills training because discussion of these behaviors can trigger urges in other group members struggling with the same behaviors. Socially anxious patients are often comforted to know that the group is quite structured and skills based. The main priority for group leaders is to teach skills. Interpersonal process issues are dealt with only when they are severe, put other group members at risk, or threaten to destroy the group's ability to learn skills. Less serious behaviors are usually tolerated, and trainers respond as if patients are collaborating even when they are not. If a problematic behavior such as not completing homework continues, patients are asked to work with their individual clinician to understand the function of the behavior and to find more skillful ways to address the issues prompting the behavior.

When a patient is involved in a DBT skills group, it is helpful for the clinician to clarify with group leaders what expectations they have of the individual clinician. In standard DBT, it is expected that individual clinicians will be available to their patients outside of scheduled appointments and that the care of a suicidal patient will be transferred to the individual clinician as quickly as possible. In DBT, a skills trainer will expect to be able to call the individual clinician when crises arise and will ask for instructions on how to proceed, with the expectation that the individual clinician will take over the patient's care as soon as possible, within reason. Additional expectations of individual clinicians in DBT include the following:

- Helping the patient develop a distress tolerance plan using DBT distress tolerance skills and identifying the pros and cons of using distress tolerance skills versus using suicide/self-harm or impulsive behaviors

- Completing a chain analysis when a patient has self-harmed and helping the patient to find more skillful ways to deal with both their distress and the problem that prompted the distress

- Working on any patient behaviors that interfere with the patient's benefiting from group skills training
- Coaching the patient on use of DBT skills in everyday life

Free-standing DBT skills groups may have all or none of the above expectations regarding an individual clinician who is following a patient attending group. Skills clinicians will likely expect that at a minimum, individual clinicians will demonstrate an interest in the skills that the patient is learning in group and will help the patient use those skills to solve the problems of everyday living. An easy way for the clinician to help a patient apply DBT skills is to have the patient briefly teach the clinician what the patient has learned each week in the DBT skills group.

It is important for individual clinicians to know that missing four sessions in a row of DBT skills group will usually result in a patient being discharged from the group. This expectation is not suspended even when a patient is hospitalized. A patient is expected to behave in such a way that inpatient staff will be comfortable letting the patient out on a pass to attend the weekly DBT skills training group.

Key Points

- Keeping in mind the myths about BPD and the DBT assumptions can help clinicians increase empathy toward patients. Reviewing the DBT assumptions with patients can be useful to set a framework for how the treatment relationship works.

- The clinician can improve the therapeutic alliance through the following: providing psychoeducation about BPD; being active, open, and direct when communicating with the patient; providing validation; working on here-and-now problems; following a structure to increase consistency and confidence; and being available between sessions.

- Self-disclosure within personal limits can be useful as a teaching tool and can increase trust and openness between the patient and clinician.

- Brief irreverent statements can be used to gently nudge a patient "off balance" when they are particularly stuck or hopeless. Irreverence can be used in GPM to lighten the emotional tone of a topic so it can be more easily reflected on and managed.

- Discussing the BPD diagnosis and providing psychoeducation about etiology, treatment, and prognosis can instill hope and have been shown to improve BPD symptoms even before therapy has started.

- In the first session, it is useful to discuss treatment duration and frequency and to explain that treatment will continue if it proves to be helpful.

- The main goal of treatment is to help the patient build a life worth living. Working with a patient to develop life-worth-living goals provides a focus for treatment. Stopping self-harm, substance use, disordered eating behaviors, and other problematic behaviors is viewed as an important step toward building a life worth living.

- Treatment contracts outlining clinician and patient expectations provide guidelines for treatment. There may be times where both clinician and patient will step outside of the framework. Having a framework provides a cue to discuss these deviations and to help get the treatment back on track.

- Having a consistent structure and approach to follow within sessions creates consistency and predictability for both clinician and patient.

- A key strategy in all effective treatments for BPD is to help patients make connections between current life events and their emotions, thoughts, and behaviors. Chain analysis is a useful strategy for making these connections.

- Clinicians need to be active in sessions and need to encourage patients to be active participants. The main focus of a DBT or GPM session is on current problems of day-to-day living, similar to what is done in case management.

- In addition to individual sessions, patient participation in any type of structured group (e.g., DBT skills group, interpersonal group, support group, drug or alcohol recovery group) is highly recommended. When a patient is involved in a DBT skills group, the clinician should speak to the group leaders regarding their expectations of the individual clinician.

—————— ●●● ——————

References

American Psychiatric Association: Diagnostic and Statistical Manual of Mental Disorders, 5th Edition. Arlington, VA, American Psychiatric Association, 2013

Gunderson JG: Borderline Personality Disorder. Washington DC, American Psychiatric Press, 1984

Gunderson JG, Links PS: Handbook of Good Psychiatric Management for Borderline Personality Disorder. Washington, DC, American Psychiatric Publishing, 2014

Gunderson JG, Frank AF, Ronningstam EF, et al: Early discontinuance of borderline patients from psychotherapy. J Nerv Ment Dis 177(1):38–42, 1989

Linehan MM: Cognitive-Behavioral Treatment of Borderline Personality Disorder. New York, Guilford, 1993, pp 376–393

Waldinger RJ, Gunderson JG: Completed psychotherapies with borderline patients. Am J Psychother 38(2):190–202, 1984

Zanarini MC, Frankenburg FR: A preliminary randomized trial of psychoeducation for women with borderline personality disorder. J Pers Disord 22(3):284–290, 2008

Zanarini MC, Conkey LC, Temes CM, Fitzmaurice GM: Randomized controlled trial of Web-based psychoeducation for women with borderline personality disorder. J Clin Psychiatry 79(3), 2018

4

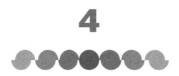

Helping in a Crisis

Support for Patients and Clinicians

Deanna Mercer, M.D., FRCPC

Anne K.I. Sonley, J.D., M.D., FRCPC

Lois W. Choi-Kain, M.D., M.Ed.

In this chapter we outline principles to guide treatment when patients with borderline personality disorder (BPD) present in crisis. This chapter will cover approaches to self-harm and suicidal behavior, intersession contact with patients, and the use of hospitalization. In addition clinician supervision is recommended and suggestions are provided around best to involve multiple treaters in patient care.

Helping Patients Through a Crisis

Self-Harm, Suicidal Behavior, and Safety Planning

According to both dialectical behavior therapy (DBT) and good psychiatric management (GPM), self-harm behavior is regarded as a maladaptive coping mechanism used to reduce distress. Studies have shown that negative affect and arousal are reduced by self-injury proxies in laboratory settings (Klonsky 2007; Reitz et al. 2015). The problem with self-harm is that although it can be helpful at reducing distress in the short term, it is not an effective way to reduce distress in the long term. Similarly, suicidal thoughts and behaviors are thought to occur in response to distress and often also serve as a way to avoid negative emotions. Self-harm and suicidal behaviors can result in obvious medical complications, but they also can add stress in relationships when the patient needs support the most.

Both DBT and GPM give detailed guidance on the management of self-harm and suicidal behaviors. The majority of these suggestions are the same, but there are a few important differences. In DBT, treatment does not proceed until the patient has made a clear commitment to the goal of putting self-harm and suicidal behaviors on hold. Clinicians sometimes irreverently explain the importance of this commitment to patients by saying, "You can't do DBT if you're dead." DBT acknowledges that patients will often be ambivalent, and the patients' commitment to putting self-harm and suicidal behaviors on hold may not be as strong as clinicians would like. In practice, however, a clinician will accept a patient committing to "do everything humanly possible" to put self-harm and suicidal behavior on hold from week to week.

In GPM, patients are asked to put self-harm and life-threatening behavior on hold while they are in treatment, and it is hoped that they agree to do so. However, if self-harm does not present an immediate or serious health risk, patients are not required to focus on it as a major goal in treatment. When self-harm does occur, the reason for the behavior is explored, and the clinician helps the patient develop other ways of coping with the painful emotions that precede self-harm. In cases in which the suicidality and self-harm are not a priority on the patient's agenda for goals in the treatment, the GPM clinician can choose to continue to work with the patient so long as the patient and the patient's significant others understand and accept that self-harm increases the risk of eventual suicide. In more medically serious or dangerous cases, a clinician may choose to consult with other clinicians, who may agree that more effective treatment options are not available. If it is within the clinician's own personal limits, these measures of informing the patient and their family about risks and benefits of addressing self-destructive behavior and of exploring second opinions can allow for treatment to continue under the agreement that the patient is adequately informed about the risks.

Both DBT and GPM communicate an expectation that suicidal behaviors should improve with treatment. In DBT, until improvement occurs, self-harm and suicidal behaviors are the primary focus of treatment. DBT does not give a timeline for how quickly these behaviors should improve but acknowledges that continuation of serious suicidal behavior is likely to strain a clinician's limits. In GPM, based on findings of longitudinal research, suicidal behaviors are expected to be among the first areas of improvement (Zanarini et al. 2007), generally improving within the first 2–6 months. If improvement does not occur, the clinician should raise concerns about the effectiveness of treatment.

DBT and GPM describe similar approaches for responding to a patient in crisis. Both approaches encourage the following: assessing suicide risk, clarifying precipitants, validating, problem solving, encouraging noticing and tolerating difficult emotions, reducing access to means, hospitalizing reluctantly, and discussing the event with colleagues.

In DBT, clinicians are continually assessing for risk of suicide. Patients rate intensity of suicide and self-harm urges daily on a scale from 0 to 5 on a diary card (see Chapter 5, "Dialectical Behavior Therapy Tool Kit"). At the beginning of each individual session, the clinician explicitly asks whether the patient has made any suicide attempts over the past week or is currently experiencing high-risk suicidal ideation or urges. If present, these are a primary target of the individual session. Self-harm is given the same priority as suicidal behaviors.

In DBT, patients develop a distress tolerance plan and a crisis plan. A distress tolerance plan consists of distress tolerance skills that the patient finds helpful when distressed; examples include using ice, exercising, breathing, distraction, self-soothing, or calling the clinician for coaching. The crisis plan includes names and contact numbers of significant others, clinicians, and pharmacotherapists; a list of all medications; a history of past suicide attempts; and the current treatment plan. This plan is intended for the clinician to use when the patient is considered to be at imminent risk of harm. When the risk of suicide is assessed to be high, the clinician is advised to involve significant others, including other clinicians. It is important to note that in DBT, patients are asked to contact the clinician for coaching before self-harm or suicidal behavior occurs, but they are instructed not to contact the clinician within 24 hours after these behaviors to avoid reinforcing suicide and self-harm behaviors.

GPM does not require that patients fill in a structured diary card. Instead, patients are asked to develop a personal method of rating emotional distress and discussing thoughts of suicide. The clinician makes explicit that the patient needs to tell the clinician when feeling suicidal because the clinician is not omniscient. Although a clinician may not routinely ask about suicidal ideation or urges, a GPM clinician always responds to any suggestion of suicide by expressing concern for the patient and assessing the level of danger. Suicidality and self-harm are not insistently discussed, however, because patients can inadvertently be taught to express their distress and despair in these terms rather than in more relatable ways to which others in the patient's life (besides the clinician) can more realistically respond.

In GPM, a safety plan starts with identifying situations, particularly interpersonal situations, and typical experiences associated with suicidal behaviors. The safety plan includes distress tolerance and self-soothing activities, and patients are explicitly encouraged to reconnect with supportive people. GPM highlights that patients need to advise friends and family that they are not required to act as clinicians and teaches patients that connecting with supportive others is centered around expressing needs directly and enlisting company in joint activities that are mutually bonding and enjoyable. The patients are also asked to identify people whom they should not seek out in crises because interactions with these specific people may predictably aggravate the patients' distress. Patients may be encouraged to contact the clinician, depending on clinician availability. The crisis plan also includes other professional resources, such as crisis lines and going to the emergency room if needed (see Appendix C for a sample crisis plan).

In both DBT and GPM, at the session following the crisis, the clinician assesses what prompted the crisis and suggests alternative ways for the patient to respond in the future. In GPM, the patient is asked to consider the negative effects of suicidal behavior, including the impact on the clinician. The clinician should consider whether their own behavior may be contributing to the patient's suicidality. In GPM, the clinician will focus on interpersonal stressors that may have precipitated the patient's crisis. Common examples of stressors include loneliness, rejection, conflict, or a step-down in care. The clinician will actively interpret how behavior during the crisis may have provided relief, in particular the perception of being cared for.

Both GPM and DBT acknowledge that clinicians are not omnipotent in their ability to prevent a patient's suicide. If a suicide does occur, DBT and GPM recommend that the clinician inform authorities and ensure that documentation, particularly from the last session with the patient, is up to date. Both DBT and GPM acknowledge that although doing so is difficult, it is important that the clinician contact the family, offering comfort and sharing what the clinician knows. The clinician also reviews the events leading up to the suicide with other health care providers involved with the patient. Clinicians are encouraged to get support from colleagues and consider obtaining consultation from a knowledgeable colleague. GPM also encourages clinicians to realize that patient suicide is an experience that "comes with the territory" and encourages clinicians to be forgiving of themselves while also being willing to learn from the experience.

Intersession Contact

Access to the primary clinician outside regularly scheduled appointments is a requirement in standard DBT. Linehan (1993), the developer of DBT, states that "suicidal patients must be told they can call their clinicians at any time—night or day, work days or holidays if necessary. A high-risk suicidal patient must be given a phone number where she can reach her clinician at home" (p. 503). However, Linehan does provide some flexibility in this requirement, allowing clinicians to limit access if they arrange access to other professional care. Standard DBT, as it has been evaluated in randomized controlled trials (Stoffers et al. 2012), generally offers individual coaching for patients on a 24/7 basis, using a clinician available by pager. The reason for providing this access is to ensure that patients are able to use the skills they are learning in DBT in their life outside treatment, particularly at times when they are most at risk of harming themselves.

DBT has rules related to phone calls: patients must call before they self-harm, and they are not to call for 24 hours after self-harming. Phone calls usually last 10–20 minutes and are not "psychotherapy on the phone"; rather, they provide an opportunity for in vivo skills coaching. Patients are allowed to make calls for three reasons: crisis coaching, skills coaching, or addressing a rupture in the therapeutic alliance. Clinicians are required to monitor the limits with respect to phone calls, address these limits in session, and if necessary place limits on the frequency of phone calls.

DBT recommends that the clinician follow up on a phone call at the next session, including talking about how the patient requested help and how the clinician felt as a result. Because a goal of treatment is for patients to be able to use skills independently and for patients to be able to effectively ask for help in their environment, by the midpoint of treatment, coaching calls are often no longer necessary.

In the GPM model, clinicians are not expected to be available at all times but are expected to address their availability with the patient. The patient needs to feel that the GPM clinician is receptive to important communications from the patient, but GPM does not require that the clinician be available 24/7. A central paradox in GPM is that the clinician wants to be called rather than have the patient make a suicide attempt, but at the same time, the clinician knows that depending on another person for safety is not an adequate or reliable plan. Because crises are expected, the patient must be fully informed about what emergency services are available 24/7 and how to access these services. It is important that this information be incorporated into the patient's safety plan. A clinician who will be away for an extended period of time may permit patient contacts by phone or e-mail if this does not interfere with the clinician's plans, or the clinician may arrange coverage if a patient wants it.

GPM suggests that clinicians may inadvertently reinforce the need for 24/7 availability by inviting patients' calls when not in crisis, offering prolonged supportive listening during calls, or failing to follow up on calls at the next appointment. GPM highlights that intolerance of aloneness is a common reason for patients' calls, and clinicians need to identify this as an understandable prompting event for distress and help patients find ways to cope with feelings of loneliness. Clinicians need to let patients know that for their safety it is unwise to be dependent on the availability of the clinician, and crisis plans need to include other supportive people the patient can call, as well as the local crisis line number and other professional supports. This maneuver is expressly designed to empower patients to rely on tools they have at their disposal, rather than relying on others in an idealizing way to be all knowing and always available.

Although most patients use clinician intersession availability sparingly or not at all, some patients press for intersession contact beyond the limits that the clinician has established, with about 15% of patients (estimated from clinical experience) calling repeatedly when not in crisis. At the appointment following each call, the clinician needs to explore the events surrounding the call, discuss the impact that the call had on the clinician, and set limits on these calls. When a patient seeks greater clinician availability, this is an opportunity for a fruitful discussion about the patient's interpersonal sensitivity and intolerance of aloneness (Gunderson and Links 2014). Although a patient may struggle with a clinician's limits, the clinician must maintain the limits while not taking the patient's desire to have more contact personally. This struggle to make contact and test the limits is best understood as a demonstration of the underlying difficulties with interpersonal sensitivity. When a patient fails to use intersession contact when it is indicated— for example, by not calling during a crisis—this is also explored in the next session, and the patient should be encouraged to call the clinician next time a crisis occurs.

In clinical environments that do not have large clinical teams, providing 24/7 clinician availability to patients can be difficult. The GPM approach to intersession availability is feasible for most clinical settings because it recommends that clinicians take into account both work constraints and their personal limits when deciding on their availability. This approach also teaches patients that other people cannot always be helpful, consistent, and available.

Use of Hospitalization

Both DBT and GPM take the stance that hospitalization should be avoided when possible. Both stress that hospitalization should be considered only when risk of suicide is high or when self-harm results in serious medical complications. A common scenario for hospitalization is when the patient is judged to be at an acute on chronic risk for suicide that calls for safe asylum until the acuity of the suicide risk returns to the long-term baseline level of risk (Zaheer et al. 2008).

GPM highlights that risks of hospitalization can include avoidance of current life stressors, including loneliness and interpersonal conflict. DBT emphasizes that hospitalization may reinforce the same behaviors (e.g., suicidality) that it is intended to prevent. If admissions are needed, short admissions (e.g., less than 72 hours) are preferred so that the patient's life outside the hospital is not greatly disrupted and so that life outside the hospital and treatment remain the priority.

Both treatments identify situations in which hospitalization may be useful. According to GPM, hospitalization might be useful under these conditions:

- Treatment reevaluation: Occasionally, if the patient is deteriorating and is presenting a significant risk to self, hospitalization may serve as a conduit to a more intense rehabilitation program, such as substance rehabilitation.

- Situational stressors: A patient may require a brief hospitalization to address a situational crisis that is leading to significant instability (e.g., homelessness, loss of a significant other).

- Shameful disclosures: Patients often struggle with disclosing important failures or secrets in outpatient therapy. These issues can include dropping out of school, losing a job, substance use, serious financial difficulty, or suffering in an abusive relationship. When the patient is in a self-destructive process of avoiding acknowledgment of growing and serious difficulties, hospitalization may be needed for containment, support, and treatment evaluation.

DBT suggests that hospitalization might be useful in some of the following situations (Linehan 1993, p. 512):

- Escalating suicide threats: The patient is making escalating dangerous suicide threats, the threats seem to be intended to get others to do something, and the patient does not want to be hospitalized.
- Relationship strain: The relationship between clinician and patient is seriously strained, and the strain is increasing the patient's risk of suicide.
- Clinician burnout: The clinician may be at risk of burnout due to continuously high levels of patient suicidality and may need relief. Although DBT encourages avoiding hospitalization, it does not advocate that a clinician become the hospital.
- Comorbidities requiring hospitalization: The patient is psychotic or has severe depression or anxiety requiring inpatient care.
- Severe medication or substance use: The patient's substance or medication use requires treatment in a supervised setting.
- Exposure treatment: Patient requires support while undergoing exposure treatment for PTSD.

When a patient is seeking hospitalization and hospitalization does not appear to be in the patient's best interest, GPM and DBT both suggest it is best to let the patient know that the clinician believes there are better alternatives to hospitalization and that it would be better if they looked for an alternative together. A GPM clinician who is reluctant to reinforce a maladaptive pattern through hospitalization might self-disclose this dilemma, saying, "I'm willing to hospitalize you despite my concern that it will not be helpful. I will do this because I fear you will become more suicidal if I don't. Am I right about that? We would both be better off if we could find an alternative" (Gunderson and Links 2014, p. 44).

In DBT, the clinician asks the patient to use a "wise mind" when making a decision about hospitalization (see Chapter 5, "Dialectical Behavior Therapy Tool Kit"). The clinician can maintain the position that the patient is capable of coping and surviving with help, while at the same time validating the patient's right to maintain the position that he or she is not able to cope. If needed, the clinician will coach the patient on how to effectively go about getting oneself admitted.

Clinician Support

Clinician Supervision

DBT and GPM both emphasize the importance of clinician support when working with patients with BPD. In standard DBT, clinician support or clinician supervision has a structured format. Clinicians meet weekly with other DBT clinicians to discuss cases they need help with. This "consultation team" is run with DBT principles in mind, and clinicians provide each other with validation and problem-solving suggestions. It is suggested that these groups have a minimum of three members. In GPM, consultations with other clinicians—either clinician-to-clinician discussions or formal consultations—are also encouraged. Thinking as a team or with the feedback of others is encouraged in GPM, but the format is flexible to accommodate what is available in the clinician's work environment.

Involvement of Other Professionals

Both GPM and DBT insist on clear roles for clinicians and expect that each patient will have a primary clinician. However, treatment of patients with BPD may also call for an array of treatment methods. There can be value in the patient's use of different providers for different aspects of care. For example, one clinician may address a particular intervention (e.g., medication), whereas another may address a different intervention or need (e.g., skills training).

GPM identifies the following advantages of encouraging a patient to work with more than one clinician or therapeutic resource: 1) the patient becomes reliant on more than one source of support, thus diluting the transference response to any one clinician; 2) having multiple clinicians lessens the risk of clinician burnout; and 3) a patient's connection to their community can be enhanced, for example, by attending an Alcoholics Anonymous or Narcotics Anonymous group.

Although *splitting*, in which a patient sees one clinician as "all good" and another as "all bad," can occur, this usually can be managed when open communication between the clinicians is established as part of the treatment contract with the patient (Links et al. 2016). GPM encourages the primary clinician not to accept the vilification of other treaters. Patients are encouraged to voice their complaints directly to other treaters. GPM also highlights that involving other clinicians may not be therapeutic when one treater fails to stay in touch with the other treater or when the treaters are unable to work together without hostility and dysfunction. In these situations, it may not be in the patient's interest to continue to see both treaters.

In contrast, DBT views splitting as a failure of synthesis of dialectical tensions between staff members rather than as the "patient's problem." Linehan (1993) suggests that treaters tend to vacillate between two poles of a dialectic: the "patient-as-fragile" pole and the "let's-get-tough" pole. Commonly, from the patient's point of view, a treater who is leaning toward the "patient-as-fragile" pole is seen as the "good guy" and the treater who is leaning toward the "let's-get-tough" pole is seen as the "bad guy." DBT encourages treaters to try to search for a synthesis between the "gentle" and "tough" positions.

The common elements between the two approaches are that clinicians need to be able to tolerate their patients being angry at them and other treaters, validate what is valid about the patient's concerns, and avoid vilifying other treaters.

GPM and DBT differ somewhat in their approaches to contact between treaters. GPM advocates that clinicians who are involved in a patient's care talk to each other directly. DBT's approach, called "consultation to the patient," is intended to empower the patient and reduce miscommunication. A DBT clinician does not communicate with other treatment providers if a patient is able to do this for themselves. This approach also applies to communication with family members, significant others, and any other individual who makes a demand of the patient (e.g., college admissions officer, human resources professional). In consultation to patients, the clinician assists patients to 1) take care of themselves, 2) convey information about themselves to others, 3) advise others about what they want, and 4) make changes in their own environments. In the situation where direct communication between treaters is required, DBT prefers that the patient also be present. Exceptions to the consultation to the patient approach are appropriate when patients are unable to self-advocate. For example, if a patient needs a letter for disability insurance or is at imminent risk of serious harm to self or others, a clinician may call someone on the patient's crisis plan if needed. In such a case, information is provided on a need-to-know basis and any information that would embarrass or humiliate the patient is kept confidential.

It is important to note that the consultation to the patient approach is also often used by clinicians providing either freestanding or skills-only DBT groups. For example, if an individual clinician would like to know about a patient's progress in a DBT skills training group, the group leader might encourage patient involvement by asking to meet with the clinician and patient via teleconference to discuss the patient's progress.

Key Points

- Self-harm and suicidal behavior are viewed as coping mechanisms that occur in the context of emotional distress and interpersonal rejection.

- It is important for the clinician to work with the patient to identify common patterns that lead to self-harm and suicidal behavior and to determine the function of these behaviors.

- It is important for the clinician to make a plan with the patient for alternative coping strategies that can be used when the patient is distressed and to let a patient know in advance how the clinician will react when concerned about the patient's risk of suicide.

- Intersession contact supports patients as they find new ways to cope in crisis situations. Intersession availability depends on the clinician's limits and should be discussed with the patient in advance. It is important to highlight to a patient that relying on the clinician as the main way to prevent suicide is not feasible. Misuse of intersession contact is rare, and when it occurs, it is addressed at the next appointment.

- Because hospitalization may become a way of dodging difficulties, it is to be avoided whenever possible. When a patient insists on being hospitalized, and the clinician does not believe it will be helpful, it is recommended that the clinician describe to the patient why hospitalization is unlikely to be helpful but also emphasize the patient's freedom to choose to be hospitalized. It can be helpful for the clinician to suggest working together to figure out an alternative to hospitalization. Hospitalization is appropriate when the patient's condition acutely deteriorates and they cannot manage safely as an outpatient.

- Having clinician supervision in some form is strongly recommended for a clinician who is working with patients with BPD.

- Having multiple treaters involved in a patient's care is not uncommon. It is important to outline clear roles as well as maintain open communication between the patient and all treaters involved.

- If a patient is frustrated with a treater, it is important for the treater to tolerate this and validate what is valid about the patient's concerns. It is also important to avoid vilification of other treaters.

- It can be helpful to have the patient involved in communication between treaters to increase transparency and to encourage the patient to self-advocate.

———————— ●●● ————————

References

Gunderson JG, Links P: Handbook of Good Psychiatric Management for Borderline Personality Disorder. Washington, DC, American Psychiatric Publishing, 2014

Klonsky ED: The functions of deliberate self-injury: a review of the evidence. Clin Psychol Rev 27(2):226–239, 2007

Linehan MM: Cognitive-Behavioral Treatment of Borderline Personality Disorder. New York, Guilford, 1993

Links P, Mercer D, Novick J: Establishing a treatment framework and therapeutic alliance, in Integrated Treatment for Personality Disorder: A Modular Approach. Edited by Livesley WJ, Dimaggio G, Clarkin JF. New York, Guilford, 2016, pp 101–122

Reitz S, Kluetsch R, Niedtfeld I, et al: Incision and stress regulation in borderline personality disorder: neurobiological mechanisms of self-injurious behavior. Br J Psychiatry 207(2):165–172, 2015

Stoffers JM, Völlm BA, Rücker G, et al: Psychological therapies for people with borderline personality disorder. Cochrane Database Syst Rev (8):CD005652, 2012

Zaheer J, Links PS, Liu E: Assessment and emergency management of suicidality in personality disorders. Psychiatr Clin North Am 31(3):527–543, viii–ix, 2008

Zanarini MC, Frankenburg FR, Reich DB, et al: The subsyndromal phenomenology of borderline personality disorder: a 10-year follow-up study. Am J Psychiatry 164:929–935, 2007

5

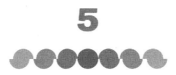

Dialectical Behavior Therapy Tool Kit

Shelley McMain, Ph.D., C.Psych.

Anne K.I. Sonley, J.D., M.D., FRCPC

This chapter is not intended as an exhaustive discourse on dialectical behavior therapy (DBT) strategies but instead is meant to provide an accessible overview of some of the techniques commonly used in DBT that can be incorporated into good psychiatric management when working with patients with borderline personality disorder (BPD). For a more extensive overview of DBT, see *Cognitive-Behavioral Treatment of Borderline Personality Disorder* (Linehan 1993). For more detail on DBT skills and useful handouts, see the *DBT Skills Training Manual*, Second Edition (Linehan 2015).

Dialectical Focus on Acceptance and Change

In DBT, clinicians are encouraged to maintain a dialectical balance between strategies that encourage change and those that convey acceptance and validation. This dialectical approach is highlighted in DBT's fundamental assumptions about patients (see Table 3–2 in Chapter 3, "Basics of Good Psychiatric Management and Dialectical Behavior Therapy Treatment"). For example, the assumption "People with BPD are doing the best that they can" suggests acceptance, while at the same time there is a push for change in the assumption "People with BPD need to do better, try harder, and be more motivated to change." The dialectical approach is also evident in this assumption: "People with BPD may not have caused all of their own problems [acceptance], but they have to solve them anyway [change]." At the core of DBT practice, clinicians move flexibly between acceptance-oriented strategies and change-oriented strategies in responsive attunement to a patient's experience in any moment within a session. Examples of change-oriented strategies include problem assessment and problem solving, exposure-based procedures, cognitive modification, skills training, commitment strategies, contingency management, and other therapeutic techniques designed to promote change.

Clinicians demonstrate acceptance of patients through active nonjudgmental listening, reflecting, and highlighting the wisdom in a patient's experience. One way of expressing validation is by communicating that someone's emotions, behaviors, or thoughts make sense and are understandable within the current context. For example, if a clinician is 10 minutes late for an appointment with a patient and the patient appears irritated, the clinician might say a validating thing such as, "I'm sorry I'm so late. It makes sense that you feel annoyed."

The following six types or "levels" of validation are highlighted in DBT:

1. Appearing interested—for example, when a person is communicating, listening nonjudgmentally, taking the person seriously, showing interest when the patient is expressing himself or herself through nonverbal behaviors (e.g., body language, facial expression).

2. Accurately reflecting—for example, when a person states, "I hate my mom," saying in response, "Wow, it sounds like you're really angry with your mom."

3. "Mind reading" thoughts/feelings/urges that have not been fully expressed—for example, when a person is describing having yelled at a coworker and is looking down at the floor and not making eye contact, saying, "It looks like you're feeling kind of embarrassed."

4. Explaining behavior in terms of past learning or biological factors—for example, when a person self-harms, saying, "It makes sense to me that you may be having strong urges to harm yourself given that self-harm is the method you've been using to cope with painful emotions over the past few years."

5. Validating behavior in terms of current events—for example, when the clinician is late, saying, "It makes sense to me that you're feeling

upset about me arriving late today. Most people would be upset if their therapist was late for a session."

6. Treating the person as competent (radical genuineness)—for example, when a person has revealed a "taboo" behavior, speaking in a genuine, human way rather than using jargon or speaking with a tone that is not genuine, addressing "taboo" topics in a matter-of-fact way and avoiding "fragilizing" the patient, saying, "It makes sense to me that you self-harm in your genital area. That is not uncommon in people who have a history of childhood sexual abuse."

When wanting to combine a validating statement with a change-oriented statement, it can often be useful to use *and* rather than *but*. This is because using *but* tends to discount the part of the sentence that came before the *but*, whereas *and* tends to create a dialectic. For example, note the difference between the following two statements: "I understand why you want to be admitted to the hospital, *but* I don't think it will be helpful in the long run" versus "I understand why you want to be admitted to the hospital *and* I don't think it will be helpful in the long run."

A DBT clinician works hard to communicate to patients that their responses are understandable within their current life context, while taking care not to validate elements of behaviors that are not valid—that is, behaviors that are not reasonable, logical, normative, or aligned with the patient's goals. In DBT, any behavior can be understood at some level, but not all responses are wise or reasonable. If clinicians struggle to find the valid in a patient's response, they can almost always find validity in the "why" of a person's response without having to validate the "what." Another validation pearl is that emotions are always fair game to validate. Consider the following responses to a patient's saying, "I'm afraid that I'll kill myself if I try to stop self-harming."

- Validate the emotion: "I can see you're really scared that things will become worse if you abstain from self-harm, and the research shows that engaging in self-harm actually increases your risk of engaging in suicide."

- Validate the why: "I can see why you wouldn't want to stop self-harming if you think that you'll be at an increased risk, and the research shows that engaging in self-harm behavior actually increases your risk of dying by suicide."

It is important to note that there are situations in which verbal validation may be experienced as invalidating in the absence of "functional" validation. For example, if a woman accidentally stands on someone's foot with a high heel and says, "Wow, that must really be hurting you," but does not move her foot, that comment is generally not experienced as particularly validating. In this situation, functional validation—removing the heel from the other's foot to stop crushing it—is needed. Therefore, it is important to note that actions speak louder than words, especially when action is called for.

Remembering the dialectic of acceptance and change can be important to avoid polarization when working with patients. Polarization often feels like a tug of war between clinician and patient, where the two individuals seem to be pulling in opposite directions. For example, the clinician might be telling a patient that going back to work (change) would be helpful, and the patient might be insisting, "That's impossible." Polarization often occurs when the dialectical balance has been tipped too far toward change. Noticing this tug of war, naming it, and "dropping the rope" is a helpful first step toward reducing polarization, especially when followed by shifting to acceptance and validation strategies before returning to pushing for change.

Commitment Strategies

Being committed—that is, turning one's mind fully (emotionally and intellectually) toward a cause or goal—is an important way to achieve a goal. In DBT, clinicians help motivate patients to make a commitment to change and home in on specific behavioral goals (e.g., showing up to treatment regularly, eliminating self-harm behavior). Drawing from motivational interviewing strategies (Miller and Rollnick 2013), DBT therapists help patients overcome their ambivalence about change and help build motivation to take action. People are generally more resistant to change if they feel that someone is trying to force change on them, and they are much more likely to move toward change when they are pushing for the change themselves. DBT uses the following strategies to elicit a specific commitment to a course of action and as ways of strengthening commitments that patients have already made.

1. Foot in the door: Elicit a patient's commitment to a larger course of action by asking the patient to agree to take a low-level step—that is, to do something that could be accomplished with a high level of success. Agreeing to a small step helps to create a bond between patient and clinician. Once the patient has agreed to take a low-level step, ask them to agree to take a larger step toward action. This ques-

tioning can be repeated, with the aim of having the person agree to take larger steps of action, as in the following example:

> Clinician: "What if you committed to not drinking for the next 24 hours?"
> Patient: "Yeah, I could definitely do that."
> Clinician: "Awesome! What about 48 hours? Would that be possible?"

2. Door in the face: Present a goal that would likely be quite difficult for the patient to comply with, and when the patient turns down the request, present an easier goal. For example, ask the patient for a commitment to eliminate self-harm for 1 year and if they say they cannot do it, then ask for a commitment to abstain from self-harm for 1 month.

3. Freedom to choose: Affirm the patient's freedom to choose to do something, while highlighting the natural consequences of that choice. For example, state "You are free to choose to be admitted to the hospital, and if you elect to go that route, then you will likely lose your new job and our treatment will be stalled for a few weeks."

4. Enter the paradox: Highlight the truths in life that are naturally paradoxical. For example, say "Hmm, it sounds like when you self-harm after a fight with your boyfriend, you usually feel better, and at the same time, self-harm also often prompts fights between you and your boyfriend."

5. Pros and cons: Have the patient list the pros and cons of not tolerating distress and engaging in problematic behavior (e.g., self-harm, substance use), as well as the pros and cons of tolerating distress and not engaging in a problematic behavior. Table 5–1 is a sample table for listing pros and cons of tolerating or not tolerating distress and self-harming.

6. Devil's advocate: Contradict your actual position or argue in favor of an irrational response to move the patient toward arguing for the opposite side. This strategy is particularly useful if you want to test the strength of the patient's commitment. Note that devil's advocate arguments have to be contentious enough that the patient is really pushed into a debate; otherwise, the patient might just agree. See the following example:

> Clinician: Would you be willing to engage in an experiment and eliminate self-harm for at least the next week?
> Patient: "Yeah, I can definitely stop self-harming for the week."

TABLE 5–1.   Sample blank table of pros and cons of tolerating or not tolerating distress and self-harming

Pros of not tolerating distress and self-harming	Cons of not tolerating distress and self-harming
_____	_____
_____	_____
_____	_____

Pros of tolerating distress and stopping self-harm	Cons of tolerating distress and stopping self-harm
_____	_____
_____	_____
_____	_____

Clinician: "Wouldn't it be hard though? What if something happens after you leave here and you start feeling intense anxiety and have an urge to self-harm?"

Patient: "No, I think I'd be able to handle it if it was only for the week. I can go running instead if the urge comes up."

Clinician: "Are you sure you can commit to that? I mean I think you can do it, but a week would be the longest you've gone without self-harming in the last year."

Patient: "Yeah, it'll be hard, but I think I can do it."

Clinician: "Okay, I'm glad you're willing to commit to that. Why don't we do some troubleshooting around anything that might get in the way of your reaching that goal?"

7. Extending: Attend to an aspect of the patient's communication that seems unhelpful or problematic, and then take what the patient said literally or exaggerate it even further. Note that you must convey that you take what the patient is saying more seriously than the patient does, or the patient may just agree. See the following example:

> Patient (*dramatic and threatening tone*): "I am going to kill myself."
> Clinician (*in a serious tone*): "Does this mean that we won't be meeting for our usual session next week?"

8. Lemonade out of lemons: Take something that seems apparently problematic and spin it in a new light such that it becomes an asset. Also, convey that both points are simultaneously true. For example,

state "Well, the fact that you're late for session isn't great because we have less time together today, and it's an awesome opportunity to do some problem solving around being on time in the future, given that reducing lateness is one of your goals right now."

DBT also highlights that it is important to strengthen commitments when a patient has already set an intention to take a course of action. For example, when a previous commitment is waning, the clinician can remind the patient of their prior resolution: "You're telling me that you want to end your life now? I thought that when you began treatment, you committed to closing the door on suicide for at least 6 months in order to give treatment a chance."

Treatment-Interfering Behavior

In DBT, a clinician directly addresses treatment-interfering behaviors that arise in the course of treatment. *Treatment-interfering behavior* is a nonjudgmental term describing any behavior that interferes with treatment. It can apply to patient or clinician behaviors. For example, if a clinician is on vacation and misses a patient's session, this would be considered treatment-interfering behavior because it interferes with the patient's treatment. If a patient misses a session because of being hung over, this is also treatment-interfering behavior because it interferes with treatment. The purpose of addressing treatment-interfering behaviors is not to place blame or find fault but rather to explore anything that gets in the way of the patient getting the most out of treatment and then to problem solve. For example, if a clinician expects to be away on vacation, the arrangement might be to have the patient see another clinician, to give the patient extra homework to do while the clinician is away, or to add an extra session the following week. It is especially useful to discuss the concept of treatment-interfering behavior within the first few sessions of treatment and to elicit examples of such behaviors that the patient anticipates might occur based on past experience so that problem assessment and solution generation can begin early in treatment.

Diary Cards and Agenda Setting

Individual sessions in DBT generally follow a certain structure. The clinician and patient collaboratively establish an agenda or focus for the session. The session agenda is usually established after a review of the patient's *diary card*, which contains a quick overview of how things were for the patient over the previous week. Patients are expected to monitor their behaviors daily on these cards. The cards should be personalized to the individual patient so that the behaviors tracked are relevant (see Appendix D for a sample diary card). Common categories on diary cards include emotions (e.g., types and intensity), thoughts (e.g., urges to use substances, urges to commit suicide and self-harm), behaviors (e.g., self-harm, drug use, bingeing), and use of skills. The use of diary cards has the added benefit of helping patients to be mindful of their emotions and behaviors over the week. Increased awareness promotes behavioral change (Prochaska and Velicer 1997). There are several versions of diary cards, including apps (e.g., Durham DBT Inc.: https://apps.apple.com/ca/app/dbt-diary-card-skills-coach/id479013889; POP POP LLC: https://apps.apple.com/us/app/simple-dbt-skills-diary-card/id666921665) and online versions.

After the patient and clinician review the diary card together, they create the session agenda to ensure that appropriate time is allotted to the most important issues. The session focus is organized according to a hierarchy of treatment targets. Life-threatening behaviors such as suicide and self-harm are the highest priority, followed by treatment-interfering behaviors, and then quality-of-life interfering behaviors that are relevant to the patient's goals, such as substance use, disordered eating behaviors, and interpersonal conflict. This means that current life-threatening behaviors (or treatment-interfering behaviors) and those that have arisen since the last session should be prioritized for focus at some point in the session. It is important that the use of diary cards and setting of the agenda be done collaboratively and not rigidly, preferably leaving time for items that the patient identifies as important. If a patient presents to a session in a state of emotional crisis, it may be necessary to focus on the patient's current emotional state before reviewing the diary card and establishing a session agenda.

Top 10 Dialectical Behavior Therapy Skills

In DBT, emotion dysregulation is posited to be the core problem that underlies symptoms associated with BPD. In DBT, skills are taught to help patients learn effective ways to regulate emotions and behaviors. DBT skills are divided into four major categories: distress tolerance, mindfulness, emotion regulation, and interpersonal effectiveness skills. Linehan's (2015) *DBT Skills Training Manual* contains hundreds of skills that a patient can use to help regulate emotions. Linehan explains in the manual that she drew these skills from many different therapeutic modalities. In building the skills manual, she included everything she had ever found to be helpful in working with patients who self-harm. The skills can benefit anyone, whether they have a mental illness or not.

An advantage to having a working knowledge of all of the skills in the *DBT Skills Training Manual* (Linehan 2015) is that it is helpful to have a variety of skills to draw on. That being said, in our experience, patients may find it easier to assimilate a smaller subset of go-to skills that they can master. Without this paring down, patients sometimes become overwhelmed when deciding what skills to use in the moment. In this section, we outline the top 10 DBT skills (Table 5–2) that we have found to be most popular and useful for both clinicians and patients. These include distress tolerance skills (STOP, TIPP, ACCEPTS), mindfulness skills ("What" skills, "How" skills, Wise mind), emotion regulation skills (Observing, describing, and naming emotions; check the facts, followed by problem solving or opposite action; ABC PLEASE), and interpersonal effectiveness skills (DEAR MAN GIVE FAST). We also discuss two additional (bonus) skills: radical acceptance and mindfulness of current emotions. For additional skills and useful handouts, please refer to the *DBT Skills Training Manual*.

Distress Tolerance Skills

Distress tolerance skills can help patients effectively navigate emotional crises and are useful when a patient is very emotionally dysregulated (e.g., when a patient is experiencing a level of distress of 8 or higher on a scale in which 10 is the worst distress the person has ever experienced). The purpose of distress tolerance skills is for patients to get through a crisis without "making things worse"—that is, to cope with the emotional distress in a way that is not incompatible with their long-term goals (e.g., avoiding self-harm, aggression toward someone else, substance use). These skills can be particularly useful when patients are in situations that they are unable to change. In effect, distress tolerance skills are used to "replace" dysfunctional behaviors such as self-harm. It is important to note that some distress tolerance skills act as a bridge or temporary measure that patients often need as they work toward the longer-term goal of increasing their use of emotion regulation skills to reduce emotion dysregulation in the long term. It also is important to inform patients 1) that distress tolerance skills typically do not work as quickly at reducing feelings of distress as do many of the dysfunctional behaviors that patients are working on eliminating (e.g., self-harm, substance use, bingeing) and 2) that in contrast to many of the dysfunctional behaviors, distress tolerance skills do not have negative consequences

TABLE 5–2.   Top 10 dialectical behavior therapy skills

Skill	Category
1. STOP	Distress tolerance
2. TIPP	Distress tolerance
3. Distraction (ACCEPTS)	Distress tolerance
4. "What" skills (observe, describe and participate)	Mindfulness
5. "How" skills (nonjudgmentally, one-mindfully, effectively)	Mindfulness
6. Wise mind	Mindfulness
7. Observing, describing and naming emotions	Emotion regulation
8. Check the facts, followed by problem solving or opposite action	Emotion regulation
9. ABC PLEASE	Emotion regulation
10. DEAR MAN GIVE FAST	Interpersonal
Bonus skills: radical acceptance and mindfulness of current emotions	Distress tolerance

Note.   Acronyms: ABC PLEASE=Accumulate positive emotions, Build mastery, Cope ahead and PhysicaL illness, Eating, mood-Altering substances, Sleep, and Exercise; ACCEPTS=Activities, Contributing, Comparisons, Emotions, Pushing away, Thoughts, and Sensations; DEAR MAN GIVE FAST= Describe, Express, Assert, and Reinforce and Gentle, Interested, Validate, and Easy manner; FAST=be Fair, Apologies, Stick to values, Truthful; MAN= Mindfully, Appear confident, Negotiate; STOP=Stop, Take a step back, Observe, and Proceed mindfully; TIPP= Temperature, Intense exercise, Paced breathing, and Progressive muscle relaxation.

and are more effective in the long run. When patients are in a state of heightened distress, they often need to use several distress tolerance skills and may need to repeatedly use skills over an extended period of time. The distress tolerance skills included in our top 10 list include STOP, TIPP, and distraction (ACCEPTS).

STOP

STOP is a skill that generally precedes any other skill that is used when someone is becoming emotionally dysregulated. The purpose of the STOP skill is to notice that one is becoming emotionally dysregulated and then to stop and think about what to do next, rather than reacting to the situation impulsively. STOP is an acronym to remind patients to do the following: **S**top, **T**ake a step back, **O**bserve, and **P**roceed mindfully.

- Stop: Physically and mentally "stop" as soon as you notice your emotions getting out of control.
- Take a step back: Take a deep breath and even physically take a step back.
- Observe: Observe nonjudgmentally what is happening around you and within you, without jumping to conclusions. If possible, imagine what the situation is like for others involved.
- Proceed mindfully: Ask yourself: What do I want? What are my goals? What might make the situation worse?

TIPP

The TIPP skill is especially helpful when a patient is at an emotional breaking point and the level of physiological distress is intense and overwhelming. TIPP stands for **T**emperature, **I**ntense exercise, **P**aced breathing, and **P**rogressive muscle relaxation. These four subskills are used to reduce physiological arousal. When a person is very distressed, the sympathetic nervous system becomes activated, resulting in increased adrenaline levels. This is known as the activation of the fight-or-flight response. Reducing physiological arousal, even a little bit, can give patients breathing room and help them avoid doing something they regret. TIPP skills are basically "physiology hacks" that patients can use to reduce their fight-or-flight response.

- Temperature: If a person falls into a cold lake, the body has a reflex that slows breathing and heart rate to conserve energy by activating the parasympathetic nervous system (the "rest-and-digest" system). This is especially true if the head is submerged. This evolutionary adaptation, referred to as the dive reflex, can be used purposefully to reduce the heart rate and breathing rate and to reduce distress. Different methods can be used by patients to induce the dive reflex through exposure to cold temperature. These include dipping the head up to the temples in a bowl of ice water, having a cold shower and allowing water to flow over the head, and putting ice packs on the temples. Going outside in the cold air or simply splashing cold water on the face can also be helpful to reduce distress. It is important to ensure that the exposure is not so cold that it becomes similar to self-harm, such as allowing the cold packs to produce frostbite on the skin. Also, it is important to warn patients that because the dive reflex slows the heart rate, medical advice should be sought if a patient has a medical condition that might make slowing the heart rate dangerous.

- Intense exercise: Intense exercise also activates the parasympathetic system. When someone is distressed and the fight-or-flight response is activated, the body is naturally primed to want to run away or attack something. Exercise serves to "trick" the body into thinking that the fight-or-flight action is being performed and then allows the person to take advantage of naturally produced cooling down (e.g., rest and digest) effects. Intense exercise can be easily practiced in most situations. Examples of high-intensity exercises that can activate the parasympathetic nervous system include jumping jacks, squat thrusts (burpees), or running stairs. It is important to note that exercise is most effective as a distress tolerance skill when it lasts around 20 minutes and a heart rate over 80% of age-predicted maximum is maintained. That being said, any exercise can be helpful to reduce distress, and what works will depend on each individual patient.

- Paced breathing: Paced breathing can also be used to reduce the sympathetic nervous system arousal (the fight-or-flight response) by activating parasympathetic nervous system arousal (rest and digest). Paced breathing works because when a deep breath occurs, the diaphragm activates the parasympathetic nervous system through the vagus nerve. There are many different ways to practice paced breathing. One method involves inhaling for around 5 seconds, holding briefly, then exhaling for 6–7 seconds. It is important to note that paced breathing needs to be continued for approximately 5 minutes or about 10 repetitions for it to be effective in activating the parasympathetic system.

- Progressive muscle relaxation: Progressive muscle relaxation is a technique that involves relaxing the body through tensing followed by relaxing. Progressive muscle relaxation involves tensing muscle groups as hard as possible, holding the tension for a few seconds, and then relaxing the muscle group slowly. It is similar in a way to intense exercise in that it uses up some fight-or-flight energy. Progressive muscle relaxation can involve tensing muscle groups in sequence or focusing on one muscle group at a time.

Pairing paced breathing and progressive muscle relaxation can be particularly effective; this involves tensing and keeping the muscles tense during the inhale, and then relaxing them during the exhale. Helpful cognitions can also be added to the progressive muscle relaxation and paced breathing combination. A first step is to identify likely negative or unhelpful cognitions that are increasing distress and then brainstorm other cognitions that might be more helpful. For example, for a patient who tends to become distressed when a friend does not respond to text messages, the thoughts that might cause distress could be "He doesn't like me," "I am socially incompetent," or "He's not responding because I said something stupid." Thoughts that would reduce distress would be "Everyone gets busy sometimes," "He has taken a while to respond to me before and it was okay," or "Even if he doesn't respond to me, I might be able to repair the friendship." After identifying the helpful thoughts, it can be helpful to combine them with the paced breathing and muscle relaxation. For example, one can think, "Everyone gets busy sometimes," while inhaling and tensing the upper legs, and then think, "so relax," while exhaling and relaxing.

It is essential that patients practice TIPP skills, and especially progressive muscle relaxation, when not distressed in order to be able to use them effectively when in a state of distress. It is advisable that patients try all of the TIPP skills to identify what works best for them. Some TIPP skills may be easier to use in certain contexts. For example, paced breathing and progressive muscle relaxation can be used more discreetly while sitting in class or in a meeting.

Distraction (ACCEPTS)

Distraction skills are useful when a person needs to tolerate uncomfortable or negative emotions and cannot immediately resolve a situation. Distraction skills involve shifting attention away from whatever is causing the distress to something else. Distraction works best if one throws oneself completely into the chosen distraction. ACCEPTS is an acronym used to remind people of a variety of distraction tools. It stands for **A**ctivities, **C**ontributing, **C**omparisons, **E**motions, **P**ushing away, **T**houghts, and **S**ensations.

- Activities: Engage in activities that are neutral or that prompt an emotion that is opposite to the distressing emotion (e.g., go for a run, take a shower, wash dishes).
- Contributing: Do something for someone else. People can get emotional relief by shifting their attention from their own problems and

focusing on others instead (e.g., rake leaves for a neighbor, visit a lonely family member).

- Comparisons: Put things into perspective by comparing oneself to other people who are worse off or who have suffered more. Some patients may find this comparison unhelpful and even invalidating; instead, they can compare how things are now to how they were at another more difficult time in their own life. The goal of this skill is to shift the patient's perspective (e.g., to alleviate distress about an upcoming presentation at work, compare the situation to 1) a time when you presented to an even larger group, or 2) a time in the past when you were not able to keep a job at all, or 3) other people who are not able to keep a job at all).

- Emotions: Change a distressing or unwanted emotion by harnessing the power of generating another emotion. By activating other emotions, it is possible to reduce the intensity of the unwanted emotion (e.g., listen to upbeat music or watch a comedy on TV to reduce feelings of sadness).

- Pushing away: Mentally "push away" whatever is causing the distressing emotion and leave it for a while (e.g., imagine in detail putting your emotions in a box on a shelf; go for a walk when angry with your partner to get some space; put off using drugs for 5 minutes and then repeat; plan a brief vacation [e.g., buy special chocolates and read a magazine, go for a walk in nature, sit on a blanket in the park]).

- Thoughts: Replace distressing thoughts by shifting the mind to other thoughts (e.g., do a Sudoku puzzle, solve math problems, memorize a poem or lyrics to a song, count objects, name as many countries as you can think of).

- Sensations: Appeal to any of the five senses, which can be helpful during times of distress (e.g., smell a scented candle or incense, drink a soothing drink, take a warm bath, look at pictures of nature or animals, listen to a gurgling brook or rainstorm).

For a full list of suggestions for distracting or soothing activities, please see the *DBT Skills Training Manual* (Linehan 2015). Other distress tolerance skills described in the manual include making meaning of a distressing situation, praying or meditating, repeating encouraging statements or quotes in your mind, and practicing helpful imagery techniques.

The following are some tips on helping patients learn and apply distress tolerance skills:

- Ensure that patients understand that the goal of distress tolerance is to effectively navigate emotional crises. These skills are not meant to eliminate or remove distressing emotions.

- Encourage patients to practice the skills in low-intensity situations so that they will come naturally when big problems arise.

- Brainstorm with each patient a go-to list of three or four skills they find useful for coping with distress.

- Make sure that patients do not overrely on distraction skills because these skills may end up becoming a way of avoiding experience.

- Once the intensity of the emotion decreases a little bit, encourage the patient to move to using emotion regulation skills and interpersonal effectiveness skills.

Mindfulness

There are many different definitions of mindfulness. Linehan (2015) defines *mindfulness* as "consciously focusing the mind in the present moment without judgment and without attachment to the moment" (p. 151). Mindfulness is not the same thing as meditation. Meditation can be a form of mindfulness; however, mindfulness encompasses more than meditation. There are many ways to be mindful in any situation, and one can choose to be mindful of anything. In DBT, mindfulness skills include "What" skills, "How" skills, and Noticing states of mind (Wise Mind). The "What" skills provide instructions around *what* to do while being mindful, whereas the "How" skills provide additional information on *how* to be while being mindful. Being mentally present in the current moment rather than mentally and emotionally living in the past or the future helps to increase awareness and calmness and to reduce emotional volatility. It can also reduce suffering in difficult situations, because painful emotions in the present moment often are enough to bear without also adding in worries about the future and regrets about the past.

"What" Skills (Observe, Describe, Participate)

The "What" skills refer to what people do when they are being mindful: observe, describe, or participate. *Mindfully observing* means paying attention to the current moment using the senses without adding words or judgments to what is observed. These skills could include observing thoughts, sensations in the body, the actions of other people, or one's own breath. Mindfully observing can provide some distance between oneself and what one is observing. Observing the current moment also helps people stay awake to reality as it is and can help people feel more alert and alive. For example, walking along a road and observing oneself walk along a road are experienced differently.

Mindfully describing means putting what one observes into words. The key is to describe emotions, thoughts, or sensations without adding any opinions and judgments. For example, "He raised his voice while asking, 'Why are you late?'" is a description, whereas "He got mad at me" is not a description of the facts because it involves an interpretation about the other's mood and intention. A trick to sticking to a description of "just the facts" is to notice any assumptions or conclusions being made about the facts and describe these as thoughts. For example, this statement would also be a description of the facts: "He raised his voice while asking 'Why are you late?' and I had the thought that he was angry with me."

Mindful participation involves fully throwing oneself into an activity with full awareness and alertness and without self-consciousness or judgment. It differs from mindful observing because instead of observing what one is doing, participation involves immersing oneself fully in an activity. A few examples of activities in which people may naturally participate mindfully are dancing, sports, painting, and learning a new piece of music. Although some activities are more conducive to mindful participation, a person can choose to mindfully participate in any mundane daily activity, including doing the dishes or brushing teeth.

It is important to convey to patients that humans' brains naturally wander to the future or to the past and judgments frequently pop up. Mindfulness practice involves noticing judgments and distractions and gently turning the mind back to observing, describing, or participating.

"How" Skills (Nonjudgmentally, One-Mindfully, Effectively)

The "How" skills describe how a person goes about observing, describing, and participating mindfully. The "How" skills are nonjudgmentally, one-mindfully, and effectively. The "How" skills can be counterintuitive for some people and can take a lot of practice and repetition to master.

Nonjudgmentally refers to practicing *not* evaluating things as good or bad. For most people, judgments tend to pop up automatically and frequently, and this is normal. The key to being nonjudgmental is to notice judgments and practice gently returning to the facts of what one is observing. It is also important to practice noticing if one begins "judging" having judgments!

More generally, DBT also encourages people to practice noticing judgments in daily life and replace them with descriptions. Judgments can be thought of as descriptions embedded with values or preferences. For example, if someone got a B+ on a test, this could result in the judgmental statement "I did badly" or the judgment "I did great," depending on an individual's values and perspective. Rephrasing the nonjudgmental description of this situation could be as follows: "I got a B+ on the test and I'm disappointed that I didn't score higher." It is often more effective to focus on descriptions of behaviors and consequences than to label things as "good" or "bad" because descriptions contain more specific information about the situation in addition to acknowledging feelings about the facts of the situation. For example, the nonjudgmental description "My friend is often late when we meet, and I feel frustrated" can lead to more useful problem solving than the judgmental statement "My friend is a jerk." Being nonjudgmental is not about transforming negative judgments into positive judgments (e.g., turning "He's a jerk" into "He's okay"); instead, it requires describing the facts and personal reactions to the facts.

Teasing apart judgments from facts is useful because judgments are often disguised and stated as though they were facts. A common judgment that masquerades as a description is the "I should" statement. For example, the judgment "I should have done better on the test" embeds the value "I am bad because I didn't do well on the test." It can be helpful to substitute "should" statements with statements of "wishes" or "preferences"; for example, saying "I would have liked to have done better on the test" is more descriptive. Similarly, words like *always* and *never* often appear in judgmental statements; it is rare that behaviors always or never occur.

Judgments are conveyed not only in words but also through tones of voice or facial expressions. For example, depending on a person's tone of voice, the description "You got a B+" could become a judgmental statement. In DBT, identifying and labeling emotions is a helpful method of rephrasing a judgmental statement. For example, the statement "I am disappointed about my score on the test" would not be a considered a judgment.

Patients commonly object by saying, "I need judgments; they help push me to do better." In responding to this, the clinician needs to highlight that judgments and self-critical statements are one of the least effective ways to change behavior because they usually contribute further to emotional pain and tend to get in the way of problem solving. Focusing on the facts of the situation is more effective when wanting to change behavior. For example, the judgmental statement "I shouldn't have self-harmed yesterday. I always do this. I'm the worst" is likely less helpful than a statement of the facts, such as "I self-harmed yesterday and wish I hadn't, and now I'm feeling a lot of shame and guilt."

One-mindfully means actively focusing attention on one thing in any given moment. It is the opposite of multitasking and not fully paying attention to only one thing in the moment. One-mindfully is easy to describe but very difficult to practice, especially for patients with BPD who struggle with emotion dysregulation and impulsivity. Learning to attend to something in the present moment without becoming distracted by worries about the future or memories of the past can be very difficult to do. With practice, however, anyone can increase their ability to have more control over their attention. It is important to tell people that it is likely that their attention will wander frequently when practicing one-mindfully, and it is important to be nonjudgmental and kind to oneself when attention inevitably wanders.

Effectively refers to focusing using all of one's resources in the moment and doing what one needs to do to achieve one's goals. Repeated invalidation can lead people with BPD to question whether their own perceptions and emotions are accurate. Because of this history of repeated invalidation, the fight to "be right" can become accentuated because not "being right" can feel threatening. Unfortunately, focusing on being right can be a hindrance to doing what is needed to achieve one's personal goals. For example, pursuing a lawsuit that bankrupts you and has no tangible consequences for the other party might be "right" but it might also not be "effective" if one of your important long-term goals is to continue to have enough money to provide for your family. Either course of action is understandable. However, it is useful to note that there is a choice that can be made between being effective and being right. A similar contrast is between "willingness" and "willfulness." *Willingness* is acknowledging the reality of the situation rather than fighting it, and then doing what is needed to reach one's goals. *Willfulness*, on the other hand, is the human tendency to sometimes fight against reality and refuse to do what is needed or to try to control situations in an ineffective manner. Having patients nonjudgmentally notice and label willfulness can be useful and is a first step toward choosing willingness in any moment. It is important to explain to patients that willfulness is a normal human tendency, especially when there is some kind of threat and one is feeling fear or anger. If patients notice themselves getting "stuck" in willfulness, it can be helpful to discuss what the threat would be if they were more willing.

Wise Mind

DBT identifies three states of mind that people commonly fall into. The first state is *reasonable or rational mind*, a state in which one is detached from one's emotions and thinking only in logical, practical terms. The second is *emotion mind*, in which emotions tend to dominate and may not be connected with what is logical or practical. The third state is *wise mind*, a synthesis of emotion mind and reasonable mind. This state combines the intuition that emotion mind provides with the logic that reasonable mind provides. Making decisions while fully in emotion mind or fully in reasonable mind can often lead to behaviors that seem like a good idea in the moment but are not in keeping with one's goals and values in the long run. Having patients practice observing and labeling their states of mind can be useful. Inviting patients to reflect on what they need and want from the standpoint of a wise mind can be helpful when they are making goals or important decisions.

Mindfulness skills are sometimes easy to describe but difficult to practice. Encouraging patients to practice these skills in session as well as at home is very important because these skills are the bedrock of all other DBT skills.

Emotion Regulation

When introducing emotion regulation skills, the clinician should emphasize to patients that the goal of emotion regulation is not to get rid of emotions but rather to reduce suffering and to help patients use their emotions more effectively. It is important to remember that many patients want to rid themselves of painful negative emotions such as shame and sadness. Some patients may have an aversive response to the idea of regulating emotions because they have been criticized for not being more in control of their emotions. It is important to emphasize to patients that they are free to change only those emotions that they want to change. When patients initially start treatment, emotion regulation skills often need to be used in conjunction with distress tolerance skills. As treatment progresses, emotion regulation skills tend to reduce the likelihood of patients becoming emotionally dysregulated. Our top three emotion regulation skills are 1) Observing, describing, and naming emotions; 2) Check the facts, followed by problem solving or opposite action; and 3) ABC PLEASE (described below).

Observing, Describing, and Naming Emotions

Many people with BPD have difficulties identifying and labeling their emotional experiences. Learning to identify and accurately label emotions is an important skill and is foundational to the use of other emotion regulation skills. DBT emphasizes that emotions, even unpleasant emotions, are important and serve a function. The two main functions of emotions are 1) to provide information about one's wants and needs and guide one to behave adaptively and 2) to communicate to others. Table 5–3 includes examples of common human emotions, their functions, typical precipitants, typical physical sensations, and common thoughts and action urges. A useful practice is to have patients notice and label the emotions they experience daily over the course of a week and notice the events that prompt certain emotions. When clinicians and patients are conducting chain analyses, it is especially important for clinicians to keep an emotion focus and help patients identify and label emotions.

In DBT, primary emotions are distinguished from secondary emotions. Secondary emotions are emotions that are learned or conditioned responses to a primary emotion. They are often generated by a person's interpretation of an event. For example, when someone cuts another person off in traffic, the primary emotion for the latter is usually fear because it is a dangerous situation. However, fear can be overshadowed by anger, fueled by the interpretation that what the other driver did was "wrong." Explosive anger is frequently a secondary emotional reaction underlying more vulnerable emotions such as shame or fear. Having patients attend to and notice underlying primary emotions can be helpful. Figuring out what interpretations or past learning has led to the secondary emotions can also be helpful. Once patients are able to identify their emotions, the next step is to help them use emotional information to engage in healthy behaviors that are in keeping with their long-term goals and values.

It can be helpful to have patients practice noticing and identifying the following elements when a strong painful emotion arises:

- Vulnerability: Was there anything before the prompting event that made you more vulnerable to experiencing strong emotions (e.g., not having slept, an argument earlier in the day)?
- Prompting event: Describe nonjudgmentally what prompted the emotion in one sentence (note: a prompting event can also be a thought).
- Interpretations (thoughts): Describe any thoughts you had.
- Physical sensations: Describe how the emotion felt in your body.
- Action urges: Describe what you wanted to say or do.
- Behaviors: Describe what you said and did.
- Aftereffects: Describe what happened next, including the experience of secondary emotions.

TABLE 5–3. Common human emotions and their functions, typical precipitants, typical physical sensations, and common thoughts and action urges

Emotion	Function	Common prompting events	Physical sensations	Common thoughts	Action urges
Fear (anxiety, worry, nervousness)	Behavior: Avoid danger Communication to others: Danger!	Threat to self or others	Heart racing, chest tightening, sweating, muscles tightening	"I can't handle this." "Something bad is going to happen."	Avoid
Anger (frustration, annoyance)	Behavior: Protect self and others Communication to others: Don't mess with me!	Goal being blocked Self or others being threatened	Muscles clenching, feeling hot	"I'm right." "It's unfair."	Attack
Sadness (disappointment, grief, hurt)	Behavior: Withdraw when continued action is futile Communication to others: I need support	Loss	Tiredness, emptiness	"I've lost it." "I've lost them."	Withdraw, avoid

TABLE 5–3. Common human emotions and their functions, typical precipitants, typical physical sensations, and common thoughts and action urges (*continued*)

Emotion	Function	Common prompting events	Physical sensations	Common thoughts	Action urges
Shame (embarrassment, humiliation, shyness)	Behavior: Avoid being rejected by others Communication to others: I'm sorry	Behavior that results in or might result in rejection	Pain in pit of stomach	"I am bad." "I am unlovable." "I am inferior."	Hide, avoid, repair harm
Guilt (regret, remorse)	Behavior: Avoid repeating unhelpful behaviors Communication to others: I messed up	Behavior violates own moral code	Pain in pit of stomach	"I shouldn't have done that." "I should have done that."	Stop behavior, repair harm
Envy (dissatisfaction, resentment)	Behavior: Obtain what others have Communication to others: I want that	Someone else has something you want	Muscles tightening, pain in pit of stomach	"I deserve that." "It's unfair."	Obtain or destroy what others have

TABLE 5-3. **Common human emotions and their functions, typical precipitants, typical physical sensations, and common thoughts and action urges** *(continued)*

Emotion	Function	Common prompting events	Physical sensations	Common thoughts	Action urges
Jealousy (possessiveness, clinginess)	Behavior: Hold onto what you have Communication to others: That's mine	Someone is trying to take something from you	Lump in throat, muscles tensing	"I am going to lose them." "They are going to take it from me."	Increase control
Disgust (dislike)	Behavior: Avoid harm and contamination Communication to others: Stay away	Something might contaminate or harm you or others	Nausea	"That is gross." "That is bad."	Avoid
Joy (happiness, enjoyment, contentment, gladness)	Behavior: Approach and obtain Communication to others: I like this	Getting what you want Doing pleasurable things	Increased heart rate, increased energy, face flushed	"I like this."	Smile, laugh, approach

Check the Facts, Followed by Problem Solving or Opposite Action

DBT describes a stepwise process to follow when patients experience strong problematic emotions that they want to change. The first step is to *check the facts*. Sometimes, it is the interpretation of an event, rather than the event itself, that generates an emotion. The same event can prompt many different interpretations, resulting in many different emotions. For example, imagine sending a text message asking a friend to spend time with you, and after 6 hours, you have still not heard back. If you think, "My friend works on weekends; maybe they're working," you might experience mild disappointment that you cannot spend time with the person. If you think, "This friend always answers me quickly; I hope nothing bad has happened to them," you might experience anxiety and concern. If you think, "This friend is always so slow to write back; that's so rude," you might experience anger. Finally, if you think, "I yelled at my friend last night; maybe he doesn't want to be friends anymore," you might experience sadness and shame related to possibly losing a friend. In all of these examples, it is not only the facts of the situation but also the interpretation of the facts, that prompt the emotion.

Check the facts involves nonjudgmentally considering all the facts, without interpretation, and evaluating whether the emotion one is experiencing (and its intensity) fits with the facts. When checking the facts, one is encouraged to be open to multiple possibilities and interpretations surrounding the facts. Asking oneself, "What is the threat?" can help to identify the interpretation that is causing the most distress. It is important to emphasize to patients that an emotion may "not fit the facts" and still be understandable. For example, if someone had previously been attacked by a Rottweiler and is now afraid of dogs, the person might be fearful around a friend's well-behaved Chihuahua. This is understandable given the earlier experience with a dog, and at the same time, fear does not fit the facts in the moment because the Chihuahua is not dangerous or threatening. Sometimes, the act itself of checking the facts can result in a reduction of a strong emotion that a patient would like to change.

If the patient's emotion remains unchanged after checking the facts, the patient is advised to proceed to *problem solving* or *opposite action*, depending on the circumstances. When the emotion fits the facts, then changing the facts through problem solving is one way to change the emotion. For example, if a person is worried because a new job does not pay enough to cover rent, this anxiety likely fits the facts, and changing the facts will require some problem solving. DBT provides the following structure for problem solving: 1) describing the problem nonjudgmentally, 2) identifying barriers to solving the problem, 3) nonjudgmentally brainstorming as many ideas as one can think of to solve the problem, and 4) choosing the two ideas that seem the best and writing out the pros and cons for each option.

In circumstances in which one checks the facts and knows that the emotion does not fit the facts but the emotion remains very intense, opposite action is suggested rather than problem solving. For example, the person who is afraid of dogs and experiences fear when visiting a friend's Chihuahua might be able to notice that the emotion does not fit the facts but, nevertheless, remains afraid. In this case, opposite action would be recommended. There can also be circumstances in which the emotion fits the facts. However, continuing to experience an emotion (or a high level of emotional intensity) is not effective. For example, a surgeon has a patient come in with a bullet wound. The surgeon's experience of intense fear that the patient might die and experience of disgust when looking at the wound would both fit the facts. However, if the surgeon's goal is to stabilize the patient, the intense fear and disgust might not be helpful or effective in that moment. In such a situation, where the emotion fits the facts but is not effective, opposite action is also required. *Opposite action* means behaving in a way that serves to change or shift the emotion one is experiencing. It is important to note that the purpose is not to mask the emotion but rather to actually change the emotion and that engaging fully in opposite action is important to change unwanted emotions.

One way to determine what behavior might be useful to "act opposite" is to identify the action urge associated with the emotion one is feeling and then to determine what behavior would be the opposite of that urge. Table 5–4 has a list of common emotions, associated action urges, and ways to act opposite.

Although basic patterns of action urges and opposite actions are associated with distinct emotions, it is important to help people identify their own specific action urges. For example, shame is associated with the general action urge of hiding. When a patient who appears to be experiencing intense shame presents to a session in baggy clothing and a hat pulled over her face so that she is barely visible to others, it could be useful for the clinician to engage the patient in wondering whether wearing the hat over her face might be a shame-related action urge. When working with patients to identify the specific action urges that they experience, the clinician can then brainstorm opposite actions that are specific to those patients. For example, for the patient who wears a hat

TABLE 5–4.   **List of common emotions, associated action urges, and opposite actions**

Emotion	Action urge	Opposite action
Fear	Avoid	Approach
Anger	Attack	Avoid (gently), be nice
Sadness	Withdraw	Get active, see people
Shame	Hide, avoid, repair	Disclose, approach, appear confident, make no apologies
Guilt	Stop behavior, repair	Repeat behavior, make no apologies, self-validate
Envy	Obtain, destroy	Count blessings, help others
Jealousy	Control	Let go of control, share what you have
Disgust	Avoid	Approach, be nice

pulled down low over her face, acting opposite may entail practicing sitting in session without her hat on. Acting opposite might increase the unwanted emotion temporarily, but in the long term, with time and practice, opposite action serves to reduce the emotion.

When engaging in opposite actions to emotion, the person needs to focus on body posture and facial expressions that embody the opposite emotion action. For example, people generally smile when they are happy; however, there is also an unusual biological mechanism that causes people to begin to feel happier and calmer when they smile. "Half-smiling" can be helpful when one feels angry or anxious. It differs from "faking a smile" because half-smiling involves relaxing one's face and turning up one's lips into a gentle relaxed smile that is not perceptible to others. Similarly, unclenching fists and having one's hands face outward in an open and welcoming way can also increase positive emotions. This open posture is sometimes called "willing hands." Using half-smiling and willing hands when angry or fearful are ways of acting opposite. Other examples of opposite actions to emotion include standing up straight and making eye contact when feeling shame or anxiety.

Imagine that you are presenting an important proposal to a committee, including your boss, and a coworker makes a derogatory remark about you during the presentation. You might feel angry. Feeling angry would fit the facts given that your coworker's comment might have a negative impact on presenting well in front of the committee. However, in that moment, it might not be effective for you to be sidetracked by anger if your goal is to present well. Opposite action to emotion in this situation may require changing your posture through willing hands and half-smiling, changing your body chemistry through paced breathing and drinking cold water, changing your thoughts by trying to understand the coworker's perspective (e.g., knowing that he will lose his job if your proposal goes through), and acting with genuine kindness toward the coworker if possible. Other opposite action behaviors could include gently avoiding the coworker and taking a time-out by politely excusing yourself to go to the washroom.

Figure 5–1 provides a brief summary of the suggested steps to follow when experiencing a strong emotion that one would like to change.

ABC PLEASE

ABC PLEASE is an acronym that helps to remind patients of various ways to increase resilience and reduce vulnerability to negative emotions. ABC stands for **A**ccumulate positive emotions, **B**uild mastery, and **C**ope ahead.

- Accumulating positive emotions: It is easier to cope with negative emotions as they arise when a person regularly experiences positive emotions. Accumulating positive emotions is like putting money in the bank. For example, if a person loses the last $20 bill one has, it will be a lot more distressing than if one is a millionaire and loses $20. Similarly, having a friend move away will be much sadder for a person who has only one friend than for someone who has several good friends. Accumulating positive emotions is useful because if you already have positive experiences in your life, it is easier to be more resilient when a negative event occurs. Accumulating positive emotions is also an important way to build a life that has meaning and value. It is useful for clinicians to brainstorm with patients as many small activities as they can think of that they can do in the short term that might be pleasant for them or for clinicians to create a list of possible small pleasant activities from which patients can choose. Many lists of pleasant or soothing activities appear online and in the *DBT Skills Training Manual* (Linehan 2015). Once the clinician and patient have identified possible pleasant activities, they work together to develop a schedule, and the patient is instructed to

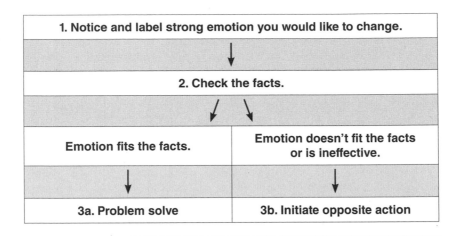

FIGURE 5–1.   Brief summary of suggested steps to follow when experiencing a strong emotion that one would like to change.

practice doing the activities on a daily basis. Patients sometimes get hung up on feeling that they "don't deserve" to experience pleasant activities and emotions. With these patients, it is important to discuss the rationale for accumulating positive emotions and to explore the shame and self-judgments that are likely contributing to their reluctance to engage in pleasant activities. Exploring whether this shame "fits the facts" and is effective is important. With some patients, practicing the skill of accumulating positive emotions might need to be framed as a form of opposite action to shame and guilt.

Identifying values and long-term goals and working toward these is another important way to accumulate positive emotions. Goal setting is covered in more detail in Chapter 3, "Basics of Good Psychiatric Management and Dialectical Behavior Therapy Treatment."

- Building mastery: Engaging in activities that are difficult but possible leads to a sense of accomplishment. Some mastery activities are not pleasurable in the moment but lead to a sense of mastery once they are completed (e.g., cleaning the house, doing the laundry). Other mastery activities, such as learning a new language, can be inherently enjoyable in the moment. Clinicians can suggest that patients plan to do something on a daily basis that leads to a sense of mastery. It is important to warn patients in advance that it is very common, and almost expected, for people to choose something they find too difficult or too easy at first and that they later need to readjust. It is also important to balance the number of pleasant activities and mastery activities the person schedules because some people tend to overschedule one or the other.

- Coping ahead: Patients can learn to identify situations in advance that are likely to be emotionally difficult and then develop a coping plan for how to successfully navigate the challenging situation. It is useful to create a "cope ahead" plan if there is a difficult situation that is planned for the future or if there is a common difficult situation that tends to recur. Asking oneself, "What's the worst thing that could happen?" and then planning for that is encouraged. Writing the plan out on paper can sometimes be helpful, and visualizing executing the plan effectively, the way an athlete does before a big game, is another useful technique

PLEASE is an acronym that helps to remind patients of the many things they can do to take care of their bodies and reduce vulnerability to emotion dysregulation. PLEASE stands for **PhysicaL** illness, **E**ating, mood **A**ltering substances, **S**leep, and **E**xercise. A person who has not slept or eaten is at a higher risk of becoming dysregulated. Similarly, physical illness, lack of exercise, and use of mood-altering substances all place someone at a higher risk for emotion dysregulation. Lack of sleep, hunger, and other elements of PLEASE frequently feature as vulnerability factors within a patient's chain analysis. Having a patient track PLEASE behaviors and work to try to optimize them as much as possible is important to try and reduce vulnerability to emotion dysregulation.

Interpersonal Effectiveness Skills

The interpersonal effectiveness skills covered in DBT were originally drawn from the existing literature on interpersonal effectiveness skills in workplace contexts. Like most DBT skills, they are helpful for most people and are particularly helpful for people with BPD. Interpersonal effectiveness can be particularly helpful for patients who have difficulties making requests or saying no to others in a direct and interpersonally effective way. It is not uncommon for patients to avoid making direct requests or to dismiss their needs repeatedly, which usually leads to a buildup of anxiety or anger and eventually leads to cutting people off through withdrawal or blowing up in anger outbursts. The core interpersonal effectiveness skills in DBT are represented by the mnemonic DEAR MAN GIVE FAST. The individual acronyms making up the mnemonic are often covered over 3 separate weeks in DBT skills groups. However, they work together to enhance effectiveness in interpersonal contexts.

DEAR MAN

The acronym DEAR, which stands for **D**escribe, **E**xpress, **A**ssert, and **R**einforce, serves as a reminder to express oneself effectively and clearly to others, especially when requesting something or saying no to a request, to increase the odds of getting what one wants. This skill helps build and maintain relationships with others. To use the DEAR skill, one first must figure out the objective of the conversation to assert one's need clearly.

- Describe: Recount the situation nonjudgmentally ("When you came home at 3 A.M. tonight…").
- Express: Articulate the emotion you are feeling ("I felt worried…").
- Assert: Ask for what you want clearly and directly ("Can you please text me next time you are going to be late?").
- Reinforce: Make clear why the "ask" is also beneficial to the other person ("…That way I am more likely to be more supportive of you going out with your friends in the future").

Note that keeping DEAR brief and to the point can be helpful to avoid confusion or getting sidetracked by other issues.

DEAR provides the content of an interpersonal request, whereas MAN, GIVE, and FAST are ways to adjust the tone and manner of a communication to fit one's objective.

MAN stands for **M**indful, **A**ppear confident, and **N**egotiate. This describes how to communicate.

- Mindful: Remain mindful of your goal and do not get sidetracked by other issues, attacks, past history, or other distractions the other person might bring up. Calmly repeating your request (assert) over and over like a broken record can be one way to be mindful.

- Appear confident: Even when not feeling confident, make an effort to appear confident through an upright posture, direct eye contact, and strong voice to make your request more effective.

- Negotiate: Be willing to discuss different options if your request is not granted. For example, if your boss does not agree to let you have Fridays off, ask to work from home on Fridays instead.

Using DEAR MAN to make requests is surprisingly effective and can be used in multiple contexts, from negotiating a phone plan to negotiating with friends, coworkers, a partner, or a boss.

When one uses the DEAR MAN skill, it is important to identify a clear objective to "assert," although that objective may be to open up a discussion on a certain topic. For example, a clear objective is presented in "Can we please talk about who is going to take out the trash next week?" Sometimes one has an objective, but obtaining the objective might not be one's greatest priority, and perhaps maintaining the relationship or maintaining one's self-respect is the top priority. Remembering DEAR MAN GIVE is suggested when preserving the relationship is quite important, and remembering DEAR MAN FAST is recommended when one's self-respect is very important.

GIVE

GIVE stands for **G**entle, **I**nterested, **V**alidate, and **E**asy manner. When one wants to ask for something from a person with whom one wants to maintain or build a relationship, asking in a way that includes the elements of GIVE is critical.

- Gentle: Be respectful and gentle in your approach, avoiding attacks, threats, and judgments.
- Interested: Show interest in what the other person is saying and listen to the other's point of view.
- Validate: Acknowledge the wisdom or reasonableness of the other person's response (see the section "Dialectical Focus on Acceptance and Change" earlier in this chapter for more information on validation). (Note that it can sometimes be useful to teach patients about the different levels of validation so they can use validation more effectively in their interpersonal interactions.)
- Easy manner: Be lighthearted in your discussion, smiling and possibly even using humor.

GIVE can be useful when a relationship is important, but it can also be helpful for patients to practice in general when conversing with others.

FAST

FAST stands for **F**air, no **A**pologies, **S**ticking to values, and **T**ruthful. DEAR MAN FAST is used when preserving one's self-respect is important.

- Fair: Attempt to be fair to the other person and to yourself and make sure that no one is being taken advantage of.

- No Apologies: Avoid excessive apologies. Apologizing when it is not warranted can erode your self-respect and be annoying to others.
- Sticking to values: Be mindful of your values and behave in accord with your personal values.
- Truthful: Be honest and truthful about what you really think or believe.

Bonus Skills: Radical Acceptance and Mindfulness of Current Emotions

Here we cover two notable distress tolerance skills, in addition to the top 10 skills we have described so far, for "keeners" who are interested in learning more. Radical acceptance and mindfulness of current emotions are two skills that are extremely useful and can be difficult to master. These two skills often do not appear useful to patients at first; however, when practiced and embraced, they can be very valuable skills for patients to learn.

Radical Acceptance

Radical acceptance means fully accepting reality as it is. This may sound simplistic, but it is often incredibly difficult to accept reality when reality is very painful. Acceptance of reality is a necessary first step to problem solving. For example, if a person does not accept that they have a learning disability, it might be very difficult for them to create an individualized learning plan or to engage in support programs that might help them reach their academic goals.

Sometimes, there are realities that leave little room for problem solving (e.g., accepting the reality of having been abused as a child). Even if problem solving is not the ultimate goal, radical acceptance remains important to reduce suffering. Accepting reality often leads to deep sadness and grief in the short term but to relief from suffering in the long term. For most people, if they do not radically accept and experience the associated sadness, secondary emotions such as anger and shame will continue to plague them whenever they are reminded of the past event, and nonacceptance then results in unresolved and prolonged suffering. Not accepting reality is akin to refusing to put antiseptic on a wound because the antiseptic is painful and then having the wound continue to fester, reopen, and not heal properly, leading to increased suffering over time.

Radical acceptance is often an ongoing process rather than a one-and-done decision. Often, a person can radically accept something one moment, and then a few moments later have the thought return that "it shouldn't be this way." Noticing nonacceptance and turning the mind back to acceptance over and over is a normal part of radical acceptance. It is also important to stress to patients that acceptance is not the same as condoning what has happened. Acceptance means acknowledging the current reality. Finally, it is important to note that a person cannot radically accept the future because it has not happened yet. One can, however, accept the likelihood that something might happen. For example, if a person is 80 years old and has never trained as an astronaut, that person might radically accept the unlikelihood of ever going to the moon.

Mindfulness of Current Emotions

The second bonus skill, mindfulness of current emotions, involves paying attention to emotions, on purpose and nonjudgmentally. Similar to radical acceptance, mindfulness of current emotions can be very difficult for patients to practice; however, it can have a big impact on reducing suffering and improving emotion regulation in the long term. Generally, if a person's primary emotions are experienced and allowed to run their natural course, they will fire, peak, and then fade away with time, similar to a wave. Patients often experience emotions as "going on and on for hours and days," and it can be important to explain that this usually happens because an emotion is reactivated over and over. The phrase "emotions love themselves" can be used to summarize this process. Often, when a person experiences a strong emotion, the mind naturally turns to thoughts associated with this emotion. For example, when sad, a person tends to start thinking about sad things, or when angry, a person tends to have all sorts of judgmental thoughts. These thoughts result in emotions being refired and maintained rather than coming and going like a wave.

Often, painful emotions, such as sadness, anxiety, or shame, are experienced as intolerable, so the wave of the emotion is prematurely interrupted and avoided using various escape strategies (self-harm, substance use, eating disorder behavior, avoidance). When an emotion is interrupted before it peaks and naturally subsides, it tends to inhibit the normal learning process, and therefore the experience of the emotion does not decrease in intensity or extinguish over time. Interrupting and avoiding emotions contributes to the belief that the emotion is intolerable. Mindfulness of current emotions involves observing the emotional wave rather than interrupting it. It can help to visualize the emotion as a wave coming and going. In the short term, mindfulness of current emotions increases awareness of the painful emotion, and this can be uncomfortable. Over time, however, the intensity of the painful emotion will decrease. An important part of mindfulness of current emotions is to notice the mind returning to thoughts about the prompting event that triggered the emotional response and then gently bringing the mind back to experiencing the sensations of the emotion itself, which allows the emotion to subside like a wave. It can be helpful for patients to practice mindfulness of current emotions first in lower intensity circumstances and then work their way up to tolerating painful emotions in difficult situations.

Key Points

Various DBT strategies can be helpful when working with people with BPD in a good psychiatric management context. These strategies include the following:

- Dialectically balancing validation and change

- Using commitment strategies

- Addressing treatment-interfering behavior nonjudgmentally

- Using diary cards and setting an agenda during a session

- Using chain analysis in a collaborative way to understand what leads to and reinforces specific behaviors the patient wants to change

- Teaching patients to use coping skills, such as the STOP skill, TIPP skills, distraction, the "What" and "How" of mindfulness, Wise mind, noticing emotions, ABC PLEASE, DEAR MAN GIVE FAST, radical acceptance, and mindfulness of current emotions

———— ●●● ————

References

Linehan MM: Cognitive-Behavioral Treatment of Borderline Personality Disorder. New York, Guilford, 1993
Linehan MM: DBT Skills Training Manual, 2nd Edition. New York, Guilford, 2015

Miller WR, Rollnick S: Applications of Motivational Interviewing. Motivational Interviewing: Helping People Change, 3rd Edition. New York, Guilford, 2013

Prochaska JO, Velicer WF: The transtheoretical model of health behavior change. Am J Health Promot 12(1):38–48, 1997

6

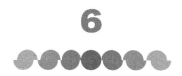

Good Psychiatric Management Tool Kit

Anne K.I. Sonley, J.D., M.D., FRCPC

Paul S. Links, M.D., M.Sc., FRCPC

In this chapter we review some principles and approaches specific to good psychiatric management (GPM), including the expected timeline for patient improvement, treatment of comorbidities, medication management, involvement of others, and focus on interpersonal dynamics and functioning.

Awareness of Timelines for Improvement

GPM provides a rough timeline for improvements that are expected to be seen if a clinician and a patient with borderline personality disorder (BPD) are working well together. This outline can serve as a framework to evaluate whether or not treatment is helping. If treatment is not helpful, then the clinician and patient need to discuss and collaborate on making adjustments (see Chapter 5, "Dialectical Behavior Therapy Tool Kit"). The general expectations around improvement, as found in the results of large-scale longitudinal studies of BPD (McGlashan et al. 2005; Zanarini et al. 2007), are outlined in Table 6–1.

Treatment of Comorbidities

GPM makes suggestions around treating comorbidities that sometimes present along with BPD. It also specifies when comorbidities should be

TABLE 6–1.   General expectations around improvement

Timeline	Improvements	Mediators of change	Red flags

1–3 weeks	Reductions in
	  Subjective distress
	  Dysphoria
	  Anxiety
		Increased support
		Situational changes
		Increased self-awareness
			Poor attendance
			Subjective distress not improving

2–6 months	Decreases in
	  Self-harm
	  Substance use
	  Risky sexual behavior
	  Disordered eating
	  Other problematic
	    behaviors
		Increased awareness of self and
		  interpersonal triggers
		Increased capacity for problem
		  solving
			Consistent disparagement of
			  treatment
			Self-endangering behaviors
			  worsen
			Activities of daily living
			  (e.g., sleep, diet) worsen
			Clinician empathy or
			  understanding lacking

TABLE 6–1. General expectations around improvement *(continued)*

Timeline	Improvements	Mediators of change	Red flags
6–12 months	Improvements in interpersonal relationships	Increased capacity to reflect on self and others	Level of self-endangering behaviors persists
	Decreased devaluation of self and others	More stable interpersonal relationships	Part-time vocational role (school, volunteer, work) not attained by patient
	Increased assertiveness		Significance of adverse interpersonal events (e.g., rejection or separation) not recognized by patient
	Emergence of a positive and dependent relationship with the clinician		
12–24 months	Improved social function	Overall decreases in fearfulness (fear of failure or abandonment)	
	Taking on school, work, and domestic responsibilities	Increased self-agency	

treated as secondary or primary. If the comorbid condition is primary, it may require specialized treatment before the clinician can proceed with treatment for BPD. Some comorbidities, such as depressive disorders, are considered secondary if they are unlikely to remit or likely to relapse if BPD is still present. Others, such as PTSD, are considered secondary if they require exposure-based treatments that can only be completed once BPD has stabilized. Bipolar I mania, severe substance use, and anorexia with significantly low weight are considered primary and should be addressed before BPD because their presence may interfere with the patient's capacity to learn. These recommendations are summarized in Table 6–2.

In the presence of a severe substance use disorder that is likely to interfere with treatment, 3–6 months of sobriety is felt to be necessary for a patient to benefit from GPM. GPM may proceed if the person's use of substances does not interfere with treatment (e.g., if a person uses cannabis daily but is attending school). That being said, the function of the substance use will likely be explored as part of the treatment, especially when a patient's substance use can be clearly linked to suicide or self-harm, interferes with treatment, or has been shown to have a significant impact on quality of life. It is also important to note that although GPM may suggest prioritizing BPD in some cases, this does not mean that trials of medications appropriate for comorbid conditions must be precluded.

Approach to Medication Management

Prescribing Medication

GPM provides specific guidance to clinicians who will be prescribing medications for patients with BPD. Although psychotherapy is the first-line treatment for BPD, patients with BPD are frequently exposed to significant polypharmacy. This is likely due to numerous factors, such as mistaking BPD for other psychiatric diagnoses such as bipolar disorder or depression, the high comorbidity of BPD with other psychiatric diagnoses, and medications being used to treat distress. When medications are used to treat distress, this often results in larger and larger numbers of medications being added over time because of lack of long-term effectiveness. The use of medication in the management of BPD is highly controversial. The United Kingdom's National Institute for Health and Care Excellence (2015) states that medications are not to be used in the management of BPD. Australian guidelines (National Health and Medical Research Council 2012), as well as a Cochrane review (Stoffers et al.

TABLE 6–2. Guidelines for addressing specific comorbidities

Recommendation	Comorbidity	Reasoning
Prioritize treating BPD	Depressive disorders Bipolar depression Bipolar II disorder Anxiety disorders Social phobia Bulimia nervosa Narcissistic personality disorder	Comorbidity will likely remit or improve if BPD does
Stabilize BPD before treating comorbidity	PTSD Obsessive-compulsive disorder Panic disorder	Stabilizing BPD first increases the patient's ability to effectively tolerate exposures
Prioritize treating comorbidity	Bipolar I mania Severe substance use disorder Anorexia with significantly low weight	These comorbidities often preclude involvement in active learning

Note.   BPD=borderline personality disorder.

2010), emphasize that medications do not appear to be effective in reducing the overall severity of BPD, although they are indicated for treatment of co-occurring disorders. The American Psychiatric Association (2001) recommends a symptom-targeted approach to the pharmacological management of patients with BPD.

The GPM approach to prescribing involves managing patient expectations about the efficacy of medications to help the patient and prescriber work collaboratively around medication management. GPM recommends focusing on building the therapeutic alliance and prescribing medications in line with what is known about their use in the treatment of BPD. Putting an effort into building a therapeutic alliance with patients with BPD almost always pays off. In the long run, the relationship with the prescriber and the messages about the role of medications in BPD may be more therapeutic than the medications prescribed.

The cornerstones of alliance building are psychoeducation, emphasizing the need for collaboration, and avoiding a dichotomous stance around medications.

Central to building an alliance is psychoeducation about BPD and how it develops (see Chapter 3, "Basics of Good Psychiatric Management and Dialectical Behavior Therapy Treatment"). When clinicians take the time to communicate this understanding, patients often feel relieved and grateful that someone understands. Once they feel understood, patients are often more able and willing to accept further psychoeducation that medications are adjunctive and empirical support for their use is limited.

It is then important for a clinician to discuss with a patient the need for collaboration when monitoring medications. Medications have a small and at most moderate effect for BPD symptoms and comorbidities. In the face of an interpersonal event that causes a wave of severe distress, any benefit may be difficult to detect, and the patient might discontinue a medication, believing it to be ineffective. Alternatively, medications that are ineffective, or perhaps even harmful, are sometimes continued. It is important to develop clear goals when starting a medication. Inquiring specifically about what symptoms the client is hoping the medication will help with is important. Having a method to monitor the impact of the medication and potential side effects is also important. The clinician could pose, for example, the following question:

> Because it will be important for us to know if this medication is helping you over the long term, would you be willing to record your anger each day on a calendar, and then we can check together to see if this is doing what we hope?

An important outcome to track is improvements in the patient's functioning. Thus, the clinician may say, for example, "If the medication helps with your anger, then the feedback you receive at work may reflect this change." Encouraging patients to read about the prescribed medications and then come back to express their concerns is also important. GPM also recommends that clinicians avoid a dichotomous stance by asserting that medications either will or will not be helpful. Instead, clinicians are encouraged to take a thoughtful and open approach: "I am not certain if medications will work. They may be helpful. It is important that we monitor."

Given that national guidelines (National Health and Medical Research Council 2012; National Institute for Health and Care Excellence 2009) highlight that current evidence does not support a role for medications in reducing overall severity of BPD, in addition to the high rate of side effects from medications, GPM advocates clearly setting a framework for avoiding polypharmacy. Prior to prescribing, the clinician should establish a policy that if the patient is failing to respond to a medication, the clinician will taper it and only then begin another medication, unless the patient is in severe distress, in which case the clinician can cross-taper.

Frequently, the main role of prescribers when following patients with BPD is systematically tapering unhelpful medications that have been started by previous practitioners. The process of withdrawing medications can be more important than starting a new medication. The clinician begins by discussing with the patient which medication would be the best one to withdraw based on current side effects or questionable benefits. The clinician warns the patient about possible withdrawal symptoms and the occasional need for other medications to be temporarily prescribed to manage withdrawal symptoms. For example, for a patient withdrawing from selective serotonin reuptake inhibitors (SSRIs), fluoxetine might be prescribed temporarily to attenuate withdrawal symptoms. Patients may have great difficulty with benzodiazepine withdrawal after chronic use, so during these important clinical interventions, patients need the clinician's time, support, and close monitoring.

When considering prescribing a medication for a patient in severe distress, the clinician communicates to the patient that although medications may provide some benefit, the most effective way to cope with acute distress is to learn self-soothing. Medications may help to some degree, but they are not substitutes for learning how to soothe oneself in the face of a crisis. The clinician can say the following, for example:

> I know from what you have told me that you are having a very tough time. I think that this medication may help to some degree. It is important that you know that skills, like self-soothing, can be even more powerful than medications in helping you to survive difficult interpersonal events.

It is important for a clinician to respond to a patient's concerns with curiosity and reassurance. This includes showing concerned attention by validating a patient's subjective reports of distress by stating, for example, "It has to be difficult to be experiencing so much suffering." In addition, the clinician can provide practical help, such as offering to be available to answer questions about medications. Given that many patients have had negative experiences within the health care system, negative attitudes toward clinicians and toward medication are not uncommon. A patient may say, "You see me as a diagnosis; you are ignoring what I am saying." Or a patient may state, "I don't want to take meds; I think I just need to change my attitude and stop being so emotional." These kinds of statements offer opportunities for the clinician to express curiosity about a patient's experiences. By responding with curiosity rather than with rejection or impatience, the clinician models an alternative way for patients to respond to their own and others' negative attitudes.

An unusual caveat in GPM with regard to prescribing medication is that at times, because the therapeutic alliance is one of the most important factors, a clinician might prescribe a medication, even if it will likely be of limited benefit, to help build an alliance with the patient. For example, it is not uncommon that patients seek help for depression and want an antidepressant, only to learn after assessment that they have BPD and are not depressed. In such a case, GPM would suggest that clinicians still might offer these patients an SSRI. SSRIs may have a small benefit for impulsivity and questionable benefit for mood instability and anger (Mercer et al. 2009); they also have a favorable safety and side-effect profile. By offering an SSRI, highlighting the uncertain benefits, and requesting that the patient monitor the effect of the medication, the clinician provides an opportunity for the patient to develop curiosity about their response to the medication and for the physician to reinforce the need for the patient's participation in psychotherapy. Thus, the clinician might say, "Although I think this may have some benefit, I am more convinced about the potential benefit from your therapy, so it will be important for you to continue your therapy."

A thoughtful and balanced clinical approach can also be helpful with a patient who appears to be severely depressed but does not want medications. If the clinician thinks a medication might be helpful, gentle encouragement is indicated:

> Given that medications have not seemed particularly helpful in the past, I understand your reluctance to try another medication. At the same time, I do think that medication has the potential to be helpful. If you were to consider trying this medication, it would be important for both of us to monitor the effect of the medication and any side effects.

Choosing a Medication

If the clinician feels that it might be useful to add a medication, deciding which medication is best will depend on symptoms to be targeted (Table 6–3). Meta-analyses of medications (Binks et al. 2006; Duggan et

TABLE 6–3.   Symptom-targeted medication options

Symptom	SSRIs[a-f]	Mood stabilizers[a-f]	Low-dose antipsychotics[a-f]	Omega-3 fatty acids+DHA[g-h]
Affective instability	+	+		+
Anger	+	++	+	+
Impulsivity	+	++	+	
Cognitive and perceptual disturbances			+	

Note.   DHA=docosahexaenoic acid; SSRI=selective serotonin reuptake inhibitor; +=possibly helpful; ++=modestly helpful.
Not recommended: tricyclic antidepressants, benzodiazepines.
Novel and requiring further research: methylphenidate for anger and impulsivity;[i,j] clonidine for hyperarousal in patients with borderline personality disorder and comorbid PTSD;[a,f] buprenorphine for suicidal ideation;[k] transcranial magnetic stimulation for anger and affective instability.[l-n]

[a]Hancock-Johnson et al. 2017; [b]Ingenhoven et al. 2010; [c]Lieb et al. 2010; [d]Mercer et al. 2009; [e]Nosè et al. 2006; [f]Stoffers and Lieb 2015; [g]Hallahan et al. 2007; [h]Zanarini and Frankenburg 2003; [i]Golubchik et al. 2008; [j]Prada et al. 2015; [k]Yovell et al. 2016; [l]Arbabi et al. 2013; [m]Cailhol et al. 2014; [n]Feffer et al. 2017.

al. 2008; Herpertz et al. 2007; Ingenhoven et al. 2010; Lieb et al. 2010; Mercer et al. 2009; Nosè et al. 2006; Vita et al. 2011) suggest, in general, that medications may be helpful for decreasing anger and aggression but have limited benefit for addressing depressive symptoms and self-harm. In the case of treating comorbidities, the usual recommendations apply; for example, antidepressants are indicated in the case of a major depressive episode. That being said, the responses of comorbidities to treatment may be somewhat reduced in people with BPD (Beatson and Rao 2013; Gunderson and Links 2008; Newton-Howes et al. 2006).

As a general rule, if patient motivation to take medications is low or if the clinician is concerned about the patient's ability to take medications regularly, the safest options are SSRI antidepressants or short-term use of atypical antipsychotics, but mood stabilizers should be avoided. When symptoms are severe and/or are having a significant impact on function, mood stabilizers and atypical antipsychotics could provide benefit. In terms of natural products, omega-3 fatty acids (eicosapentaenoic acid [E-EPA], docosahexaenoic acid [DHA]) have been evaluated in patients with BPD, and they may have modest benefit on mood symptoms, usually focusing on E-EAP plus DHA in the range of 1–2 g/day (Hancock-Johnson et al. 2017; Stoffers and Lieb 2015). Some patients will be motivated to go forward with no psychotropic medication and focus on their psychosocial interventions. In GPM, medications are considered adjunctive to recovery from BPD; therefore, clinicians should support the patients' decisions and primarily focus on withdrawing patients from their current medications.

It is important to note that in standard dialectical behavior therapy (DBT), even when the primary clinician is a physician, the primary clinician generally does not prescribe medications. The reasoning for this is based on the experience that patients with BPD who misuse prescription medications are often dishonest about their use of medications. When the primary clinician manages medication, the patient has an incentive to lie about medication abuse in order to get more drugs from the clinician.

Summary of Psychopharmacology Approach

The following takeaway points can be helpful for clinicians prescribing for patients with BPD.

1. Provide psychoeducation about BPD and the efficacy or lack of efficacy of medications in treating this population. For patients who wish to proceed in treatment without medication, validate their de-

cision, indicating that psychotherapy is the established first-line intervention for BPD.

2. Emphasize collaboration in monitoring medications, with a concrete goal in mind.

   - "What are the symptoms that you are hoping medication will help with?"
   - "It will be important for us to know for sure if this medication is helping you over the long term. Would you be willing to record your anger each day on a calendar and then we can look at it together?"
   - "If the medication works, how will it help your functioning at work or school?"

3. Avoid a dichotomous stance on medications: "I am not certain if medications will work. They may be helpful. It is important that we monitor."

4. Avoid polypharmacy. Establish a policy that, if your patient is failing to respond to a medication, you will taper it and only then begin another medication.

5. Be extra clear about expectations when prescribing a medication to someone in severe distress: "I know from what you have told me that you are having a very tough time. I think that this medication may help to some degree. It is important that you know that skills, like self-soothing, can be even more powerful than medications in helping you to survive difficult interpersonal events."

6. Respond to concerns with curiosity rather than rejection or impatience.

7. Be aware of how medication management can be used to foster a therapeutic alliance.

8. Treat comorbidities in keeping with guidelines. However, be aware that recommended medications may not be as effective in people with BPD.

9. SSRIs have limited side effects and may be helpful for affective instability, anger, and impulsivity. Antipsychotics have a more negative side-effect profile but may be helpful for anger, impulsivity, and perceptual disturbances. Mood stabilizers have been shown to be helpful for anger and impulsivity in some studies but can be dangerous in overdose and have a more negative side-effect profile.

10. If possible, consider having separate treaters for prescribing medications and acting as the primary clinician, especially in treating patients who struggle with misusing prescription medications.

Involvement of Significant Others

In GPM, involving family members in the patient's care is generally a goal of treatment. Although this effort is not always successful, many families are relieved to be included in the care of their family member, and their involvement is often helpful. If families are not willing to participate in the patient's treatment, then clinicians may have to help a patient accept this reality. Patients are sometimes hesitant to have significant others involved in treatment. However, if the patient appreciates that the objective of involving family members is to have them understand the patient better and to be more effective in supporting the patient, then often the patient is more open to this involvement.

When a patient refuses family involvement, treatment generally can proceed anyway. However, in some situations, a patient's refusal to involve family can be dangerous. Both DBT and GPM advocate for involving the family when the risk of suicide is high. In GPM, not insisting on contact with significant others is a serious mistake when a patient with serious suicide risk is refusing to allow contact with family members. Even without the patient's permission, a clinician can obtain collateral information from the person's significant others and inform the family about crisis resources. When the patient's suicidality or self-harm is occurring in relation to interactions with family members whom the patient lives with and is financially dependent on, it may be important to insist on family involvement. This will facilitate providing psychoeducation to the family to help them become allies in the patient's treatment. Agreeing to not involve the family can lead to the patient's idealization of the treater or to the patient's dismissal of the treater as a weak link.

The following are GPM strategies for involving families.

1. Validation and support: Listen to and validate the family's fears of the patient dying by suicide and acknowledge the chronic stress they are under and financial burdens they have incurred. Families bear a heavy burden, and "bad" parents are usually uninformed or ill themselves.

2. Psychoeducation: Explain to parents what BPD is, how it develops, and what the prognosis is (see Chapters 3 and 5). Highlight that their child with BPD has special needs and may not respond to parenting that has been effective with other children. Encourage families not to take their child's anger or blame too personally and to try to avoid fighting back when criticized.

3. Types of family involvement: Encourage families to be involved in support groups, conjoint sessions, or family therapy.

4. Specific guidelines for families:

- Pace of change: Go slowly. Expect change to be slow and to fluctuate.

- Family environment: Maintain routines as much as possible, and make time for chats about light, neutral matters.

- Validating emotions: Listen to your family member expressing negative emotions. Avoid saying, "It isn't so," or trying to make the feelings go away. Model using words to express your own fear, loneliness, inadequacy, anger, or need.

- Managing crises: Unless agreed upon in advance, do not ignore self-destructive acts or threats and also do not panic or reinforce the behavior. It is useful for the family to be knowledgeable about local crisis mental health services and aware of the patient's safety plan.

- Collaboration and consistency: Be as consistent as possible. Consistency across family members is also helpful. If you request something of your family member with BPD, ask if the family member thinks he or she can do what is asked. If you want to help your family member with BPD, ask if he or she wants your help.

- Limit setting: Set limits around what you are willing to tolerate and make this known in clear simple language so that your family member knows what to expect. Walk away from threats, tantrums, and violence, and return to discuss later. Do not protect family members from the natural consequences of their actions; bumping into a few walls is usually necessary when learning about reality. Avoid using ultimatums other than as a last resort; use them only if you can and will carry through.

In contrast to GPM, DBT does not have a specific emphasis on involving families or significant others in treatment; however, family involvement is still common. In DBT, the clinician is encouraged to have the patient present when involving family members and to encourage the patient to speak for himself or herself as much as possible in these interactions. In DBT, when there are difficulties in relationships with family members and these are deemed to be important to the patient, these difficulties are addressed in treatment. In the interpersonal effectiveness skills training modules, patients learn how to ask for things or say no to unwanted requests, while at the same time protecting or improving their relationships.

Also, the clinician can introduce families to the Family Connections program, a network of support groups associated with the DBT model.

These groups are available to family members, partners, and friends of people with BPD. They are available free of charge and are usually run by family members of people with BPD who have received training to be facilitators. In Family Connections, family members learn DBT skills in order to be better able to support their family members with BPD. Family Connections groups are available throughout the United States and Canada and in several other countries around the world. Family Connections is also available via teleconference through the National Education Alliance for Borderline Personality Disorder. For more information about Family Connections, see www.borderlinepersonalitydisorder.org or www.sashbear.org.

Focus on Interpersonal Dynamics

In GPM, interpersonal events, particularly those involving interpersonal rejection, are presumed to have a central role in suicide and self-harm acts. The clinician communicates to the patient that the clinician will help the patient find ways to manage self-harm and other unwanted behaviors, but to see significant improvement, the patient needs to be able to notice and manage difficult interpersonal events and build stable social supports to decrease the cause of suicide and self-harm behaviors.

The clinician can help the patient improve his or her ability to manage difficult interpersonal events in several ways. An initial intervention would be to help the patient become aware of the interpersonal events that frequently lead to self-harm or other unwanted behaviors. Chain analysis is one way to become aware of these interpersonal events (see Chapters 3 and 5). When completing a chain analysis to understand events prompting an episode of self-harm, suicide, or impulsive behavior, a GPM clinician will actively search for an interpersonal event. If a patient responds, "Nothing happened," the GPM clinician may accept this response but needs to stay open to the possibility that an interpersonal event may have been involved or perhaps that "Nothing happened" is a clue that loneliness might have been the interpersonal event. When exploring interpersonal events, it is important for the clinician to assist patients in noticing, differentiating, and labeling the emotions—commonly sadness and shame—that arise during these events.

Over time, the clinician and the patient will begin to notice patterns and interpersonal stressors that more commonly lead to distress for the patient. The clinician and patient can then work together to devise a plan on how to intervene more effectively in response to interpersonal rejection so that the patient is less likely to become paranoid, help rejecting, or suicidal. It is also important to help the patient start to experience that the painful emotions associated with interpersonal rejection can be approached, allowed, and accepted. The clinician and patient can also work together to try to reduce exposures to unnecessary interpersonal stress (e.g., eliminating unhelpful stressful relationships).

Drafting of Autobiography

Instability of self-image, or sense of self, is one of the core symptoms of BPD (American Psychiatric Association 2013). GPM suggests that helping patients with BPD to develop a coherent narrative is an intervention that can be helpful. In GPM, this is known as "making sense of yourself and your life." This narrative is developed in every session because treatment involves creating an awareness of common patterns the patient gets into and involves making links between interpersonal events, emotions, and behaviors. It also involves connecting current events to what has happened in previous sessions and at other times in the patient's life.

GPM suggests that having the patient write out an autobiography of their life to date can be helpful in promoting the development of a coherent narrative for the patient. This is generally best done as homework that can then be brought in and discussed in session. The clinician can begin the process by asking the patient to draw their family tree and explain it to the clinician or to make a timeline with significant events in the patient's life. The process is flexible and can involve as much or as little detail as the clinician and patient deem to be helpful.

Focus on Function

Patients with BPD tend to remit symptomatically with treatment, and long-term follow-up studies have demonstrated that even without intensive or specific treatment, patients with BPD have high rates of remission at 10-year follow-up (Gunderson et al. 2011; Zanarini et al. 2010b). Unfortunately, however, this improvement in symptoms does not necessarily lead to improvement in terms of functioning, such as participation in work, school, or other productive activities (Zanarini et al. 2010a).

GPM suggests that as a part of treatment, patients should be directed to develop a goal of having a productive activity, whether it is volunteering, education, or employment. GPM specifies that initial goals should be related to work rather than relationships because work helps the patient to develop an independent source of self-direction and identity, which can then help stabilize relationships as treatment progresses.

With development of a life worth living, individuals may become less prone to experiencing the most extreme stages of interpersonal sensitivity: aloneness and despair. In the face of interpersonal stress, having a stable productive activity can mean that people are less likely to seriously harm themselves or their relationships. Clinicians are encouraged to prioritize worklike activities throughout treatment. The ultimate goal would be for the patient to have a productive activity as the treatment ends.

In GPM, some of the treatment time must be devoted to setting and reviewing the goals related to having a productive activity. At the start of treatment, creating a goal can be difficult for patients, and the first meaningful achievement may be simply setting an achievable goal. The goals need to be short-term, precise, and measurable. Often, early sessions focus on the barriers to achieving these early goals. Throughout GPM treatment, the need for the patient to focus on life outside of treatment will constantly be emphasized. The patient will be reminded repeatedly that meaningful activity will lead, or has led, to the patient's having increased self-esteem, self-agency, and self-identity.

Key Points

Strategies emphasized in GPM that can be helpful when working with people with BPD include the following:

- Awareness of timelines: Monitor patient improvement; if there is a significant disparity between the patient's progress and expected timelines for improvement, discuss and collaborate with the patient on making adjustments.

- Treatment of comorbidities: Keep in mind that treating BPD will result in improvement in most comorbidities (e.g., depression, bipolar depression, bipolar II disorder, anxiety, bulimia). Remember that often one needs to treat comorbidities that will impair a patient's ability to cognitively engage in treatment (e.g., bipolar I mania, severe substance use, severe anorexia) before treating BPD.

- Approach to psychopharmacology: When managing medications, build an alliance, be clear about expectations for improvement, monitor side effects and symptoms in a structured and collaborative way, and avoid polypharmacy.

- Involvement of significant others: Involve significant others in treatment. Provide significant others with validation, support, psychoeducation about BPD, and guidelines around how to best support their family member with BPD.

- Focus on interpersonal dynamics: Be on the lookout for interpersonal rejection or loneliness as prompting events for self-harm, suicidal behavior, or other impulsive behaviors. Help the patient become aware of these patterns, find alternative ways of coping, and reduce exposure to unnecessary interpersonal stress.

- Drafting of autobiography: Help the patient create a more coherent life narrative using a timeline, family tree, or autobiography.

- Focus on function: Help the patient set a goal with regard to a productive activity (e.g., work, volunteering, school). Having a commitment to a productive activity can increase self-efficacy and focusing on "work before love" can help increase stability in the face of interpersonal stresses.

––––––––––– ●●● –––––––––––

References

American Psychiatric Association: Practice guideline for the treatment of patients with borderline personality disorder. Am J Psychiatry 158 (10 suppl):1–52, 2001

American Psychiatric Association: Diagnostic and Statistical Manual of Mental Disorders, 5th Edition. Arlington, VA, American Psychiatric Association, 2013

Arbabi M, Hafizi S, Ansari S, et al: High frequency TMS for the management of borderline personality disorder: a case report. Asian J Psychiatr 6(6):614–617, 2013

Beatson JA, Rao S: Depression and borderline personality disorder. Med J Aust 199(6):S24–S27, 2013

Binks CA, Fenton M, McCarthy L, et al: Pharmacological interventions for people with borderline personality disorder. Cochrane Database Syst Rev (1):CD005653, 2006

Cailhol L, Roussignol B, Klein R, et al: Borderline personality disorder and rTMS: a pilot study. Psychiatry Res 216(1):155–157, 2014

Duggan C, Huband N, Smailagic N, et al: The use of pharmacological treatments for people with personality disorder: a systematic review of randomized controlled trials. Personal Ment Health 2(3):119–170, 2008

Feffer K, Peters SK, Bhui K, et al: Successful dorsomedial prefrontal rTMS for major depression in borderline personality disorder: three cases. Brain Stimul 10(3):716–717, 2017

Golubchik P, Sever J, Zalsman G, Weizman A: Methylphenidate in the treatment of female adolescents with cooccurrence of attention deficit/hyperactivity disorder and borderline personality disorder: a preliminary open-label trial. Int Clin Pharmacol 23(4):228–231, 2008

Gunderson JG, Links PS: Borderline Personality Disorder: A Clinical Guide, 2nd Edition. Washington, DC, American Psychiatric Publishing, 2008

Gunderson JG, Stout RL, McGlashan TH, et al: Ten-year course of borderline personality disorder: psychopathology and function from the Collaborative Longitudinal Personality Disorders Study. Arch Gen Psychiatry 68:827–837, 2011

Hallahan B, Hibbeln JR, Davis JM, Garland MR: Omega-3 fatty acid supplementation in patients with recurrent self-harm. Single-centre double-blind randomised controlled trial. Br J Psychiatry 190:118–122, 2007

Hancock-Johnson E, Griffiths C, Picchioni M: A focused systematic review of pharmacological treatment for borderline personality disorder. CNS Drugs 31(5):345–356, 2017

Herpertz SC, Zanarini M, Schulz CS, et al: World Federation of Societies of Biological Psychiatry (WFSBP) guidelines for biological treatment of personality disorders. World J Biol Psychiatry 8(4):212–244, 2007

Ingenhoven T, Lafay P, Rinne T, et al: Effectiveness of pharmacotherapy for severe personality disorders: meta-analyses of randomized controlled trials. J Clin Psychiatry 71(1):14–25, 2010

Lieb K, Völlm B, Rücker G, et al: Pharmacotherapy for borderline personality disorder: Cochrane Systematic Review of Randomised Trials. Br J Psychiatry 196(1):4–12, 2010

McGlashan TH, Grilo CM, Sanislow CA, et al: Two-year prevalence and stability of individual DSM-IV criteria for schizotypal, borderline, avoidant, and obsessive-compulsive personality disorders: towards a hybrid model of Axis II disorders. Am J Psychiatry 162(5):883–889, 2005

Mercer D, Douglass AB, Links PS: Meta-analyses of mood stabilizers, antidepressants and antipsychotics in the treatment of borderline personality disorder: effectiveness of depression and anger symptoms. J Pers Disord 23(2):156–174, 2009

National Health and Medical Research Council: Clinical Practice Guidelines for the Management of Borderline Personality Disorder. Canberra, Australia, National Health and Medical Research Council, 2012

National Institute for Health and Care Excellence: Borderline Personality Disorder: Treatment and Management (Report No CG78). London, National Institute for Health and Care Excellence, 2009

National Institute for Health and Care Excellence: Borderline Personality Disorder: Treatment and Management (6-Year Review). London, National Institute for Health and Care Excellence, 2015

Newton-Howes G, Tyrer P, Johnson T: Personality disorder and the outcome of depression: meta-analysis of published studies. Br J Psychiatry 188:13–20, 2006

Nosè M, Cipriani A, Biancosino B, et al: Efficacy of pharmacotherapy against core traits of borderline personality disorder: meta-analysis of randomized controlled trials. Int Clin Psychopharmacol 21(6):345–353, 2006

Prada P, Nicastro R, Zimmermann J, et al: Addition of methylphenidate to intensive dialectical behavior therapy for patients suffering from comorbid borderline personality disorder and ADHD: a naturalistic study. Atten Defic Hyperact Disord 7(3):199–209, 2015

Stoffers JM, Lieb K: Pharmacotherapy for borderline personality disorder: current evidence and recent trends. Curr Psychiatry Rep 17:534, 2015

Stoffers J, Völlm BA, Rücker, G et al: Pharmacological interventions for borderline personality disorder. Cochrane Database Syst Rev 6(6):CD005653, 2010

Vita A, De Peri L, Sacchetti E: Antipsychotics, antidepressants, anticonvulsants, and placebo on the symptom dimensions of borderline personality disorder: a meta-analysis of randomized controlled and open-label trials. J Clin Psychopharmacol 31(5):613–624, 2011

Yovell Y, Bar G, Mashiah M, et al: Ultra-low-dose buprenorphine as a time-limited treatment for severe suicidal ideation: a randomized controlled trial. Am J Psychiatry 173:491–498, 2016

Zanarini MC, Frankenburg FR: Omega-3 fatty acid treatment of women with borderline personality disorder: a double-blind, placebo-controlled pilot study. Am J Psychiatry 160(1):167–169, 2003

Zanarini MC, Frankenburg FR, Reich DB, et al: The subsyndromal phenomenology of borderline personality disorder: a 10-year follow-up study. Am J Psychiatry 164:929–935, 2007

Zanarini MC, Frankenburg FR, Reich DB, Fitzmaurice G: The 10-year course of psychosocial functioning among patients with borderline personality disorder and Axis II comparison subjects. Acta Psychiatr Scand 122(2):103–109, 2010a

Zanarini MC, Frankenburg FR, Reich DB, Fitzmaurice G: Time to attainment of recovery from borderline personality disorder and stability of recovery: a 10-year prospective follow-up study. Am J Psychiatry 167:663–667, 2010b

7

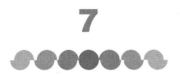

Case Illustrations

Anne K.I. Sonley, J.D., M.D., FRCPC

Lois W. Choi-Kain, M.D., M.Ed.

Four case illustrations are presented in this chapter that highlight the application of the GPM and DBT technique described throughout this book. Each case description is interrupted several times for readers to consider what actions might be taken next. At each of these decision points, questions are posed with a list of several possible response options. A discussion of the options is provided as well as ratings of the potential helpfulness and harmfulness of each option. Please note that there are sometimes multiple helpful options presented.

Decision Point Option Ratings
1=helpful
2=possibly helpful, with continuing reservations
3=not helpful or even harmful

Vignette 1: Providing Psychoeducation in the Primary Care Setting (Jacky)

You are a rural family doctor who has struggled to work with patients in your practice who have borderline personality disorder (BPD). You recently read this manual and watched the free online good psychiatric management (GPM) videos (see Appendix E in this manual) to see if they might help. Today, you are scheduled to see a 17-year-old female named Jacky, whom who followed in your practice when she was a child. You have not seen Jacky since she was 8 or 9, but you recall her to be an anxious child who used to have frequent stomachaches. During the 15-minute appointment, Jacky describes that she is leaving for college in the fall and her boyfriend broke up with her because they are going to different colleges. The breakup happened last week, and she has been feeling "depressed" ever since. She states that she hates her ex-boyfriend and feels that he was just using her. She is worried that she will gain weight because she has been bingeing on whatever she can find in the cupboard over the past week. When you inquire about self-harm, she reports that she has been cutting herself a few times a week for the past 2 years in inconspicuous areas "when things get bad." When you examine the cuts, you see that they are superficial and do not appear infected. Jacky denies any current active suicidal ideation but states that she often wishes she were dead and has had thoughts like this since she was a child. She describes binge drinking on the weekend with friends and has "tried weed a few times." She does not want her parents to know she is here.

1. What are your next steps?
   A. Start a selective serotonin reuptake inhibitor (SSRI).
   B. Book a follow-up appointment to further explore BPD, anxiety, and depression with the patient.
   C. Contact her parents despite her objections.
   D. Refer her to a psychiatrist.
   E. Send her to the emergency room (ER) because of the self-harm.
   F. Order blood work to look for other physical causes of low mood.

Discussion of Options
1=helpful; 2=possibly helpful, continuing reservations; 3=not helpful or even harmful

A. Start a selective serotonin reuptake inhibitor (SSRI). [3] In this 15-minute appointment, you have been able to assess safety but have not had the time to properly assess Jacky's mood and BPD symptoms. She reports being "depressed" for 1 week, which is not a sufficient length of time to qualify as a major depressive episode. Starting an SSRI at this point would be premature and may result in her being maintained on a medication that is not helpful to her.
B. Book a follow-up appointment to further explore BPD, anxiety, and depression with the patient. [1] This would likely be helpful to clarify her symptoms and give you time to provide psychoeducation and make a plan going forward.

C. Contact her parents despite her objections. [3] Family involvement is encouraged but not required. It is especially important if self-harm and other behaviors seem to be linked to conflicts within the family. Encouraging Jacky to involve her family can be raised again in the future as you continue to work with her.

D. Refer her to a psychiatrist. [2] You could refer Jacky to a psychiatrist for further assessment. However, it is often a long wait to see a psychiatrist, and there are several things you can do to help her in the meantime.

E. Send her to the emergency room (ER) because of the self-harm. [3] This would likely not be helpful. Jacky's cuts are superficial and do not require medical attention. Outpatient care will be more useful than an ER visit or acute hospitalization. Sending her to the ER might be useful if her self-harm is escalating in a dangerous way or requires medical attention such as stitches or antibiotics.

F. Order blood work to look for other physical causes of low mood. [2] This could be done so you have the results when you meet with Jacky next or could wait until you have clarified her symptoms further to determine if this is necessary.

You tell Jacky that you think it would be helpful to involve her parents but reassure her that you will respect her confidentiality. You book a 30-minute follow-up appointment for the following week to further explore BPD and depression with her, and you order blood work to look for anemia and hypothyroidism in the meantime. She says, "Don't I need to take an antidepressant or to see a psychiatrist or something? I'm really depressed." You reply, "We only had 15 minutes to meet today. I would like to get the blood work back and meet again to talk to you a bit more about your symptoms and discuss antidepressants with you then. I can also refer you to a psychiatrist, but it will likely take 3–6 months for you to be seen. In the meantime, let's see if we can understand these problems better so we can help you manage what you're feeling."

When you see Jacky the following week, she tells you that she and her boyfriend have decided to stay together. She reports feeling quite a bit better. She now describes her boyfriend in glowing terms and says she was just being silly last week. There are no abnormalities in her blood work. When you ask about mood, Jacky identifies with the term *emotionally intense* and describes her mood as fluctuating from sad to anxious to angry frequently. These moods last hours to days rather than weeks. Jacky does not recall a period of time in which her mood was consistently low for 2 weeks or a period of time in which she was not sleeping and had elevated or irritable mood. She does describe herself as a "worrier" and says she worries about "everything." She is especially anxious in social settings.

2. What do you do next?

A. Send her home and cancel the referral to the psychiatrist. She seems to be doing fine now that she and her boyfriend are back together.

B. Go through the criteria for BPD with her to see if they resonate with her and provide psychoeducation.

C. Discuss starting an SSRI for anxiety.

Discussion of Options
1=helpful; 2=possibly helpful, continuing reservations; 3=not helpful or even harmful

A. Send her home and cancel the referral to the psychiatrist. She seems to be doing fine now that she and her boyfriend are back together. [3] Jacky's mood has improved temporarily in response to increased support from her boyfriend; however, her emotion dysregulation, self-harm, binge eating, and anxiety remain concerning.

B. Go through the criteria for BPD with her to see if they resonate with her and provide psychoeducation. [1] From her description, it sounds as though Jacky might have BPD. Going through the printed criteria together can be an efficient and collaborative way to discuss the diagnosis and start providing psychoeducation.

C. Discuss starting an SSRI for anxiety. [2] This discussion may be reasonable but is not necessary at this juncture. Comorbidities such as depressed mood and anxiety often resolve as BPD symptoms resolve. If anxiety or depression were interfering with Jacky's ability to participate in treatment, this would be a reason to treat the comorbidity more urgently.

When you show Jacky the criteria for BPD, she identifies with them and describes how anger, feelings of emptiness, and difficulties being alone have been problematic for her. You then describe the biosocial theory of BPD, which resonates with her. You discuss her anxiety and the fact that it might improve as her BPD symptoms improve, but you also discuss how anxiety can be targeted with an antidepressant medication. She is no longer interested in starting a medication. You ask if she would like to follow up with you so that you can work together on reducing her BPD symptoms, including bingeing and self-harm, and she agrees.

You book another 30-minute appointment for the following week. The following week, Jacky reports that she and her boyfriend have broken up again, but this time "for real." She describes that she has been "depressed" again for the last 3 days and appears quite sad. She then asks for an antidepressant again, saying, "I just need something to help me."

3. What do you do next?

   A. Prescribe an antidepressant.
   B. Tell her that she is not depressed and that an antidepressant will not be helpful in this situation.
   C. Assess suicide risk.
   D. Make a connection between her jeopardized relationship and her mood.
   E. Provide psychoeducation about medications.

Discussion of Options

1=helpful; 2=possibly helpful, continuing reservations; 3=not helpful or even harmful

A. Prescribe an antidepressant. **[2]** This would require further discussion and should only be done in a thoughtful manner rather than in response to a moment of acute distress.

B. Tell her she is not depressed and an antidepressant will not be helpful in this situation. **[3]** This might be true, but without further exploration and discussion, this will likely be experienced by Jacky as an invalidating response or a rejection of her distress.

C. Assess suicide risk. **[1]** Given the change in Jacky's mood, the significant social rejection (breakup with boyfriend), and her history of chronic suicidal ideation and self-harm, it would be prudent to reevaluate her suicide risk.

D. Make a connection between her jeopardized relationship and her mood. **[1]** This is an opportunity to help Jacky make a connection between the breakup and her mood. Helping patients understand these patterns is one of the elements of effective treatments for BPD.

E. Provide psychoeducation about medications. **[1]** Addressing Jacky's question about starting a medication directly and openly will likely be helpful. It can be useful to outline what symptoms medications will and will not help with and to emphasize the need to have specific goals that can be monitored when starting a medication.

You say, "Wow, I would be sad too if an important relationship was ending." You then describe how antidepressant medications are mainly helpful for continuous low mood and require a few weeks to work. They do not provide instantaneous relief. You describe that they might be particularly helpful if taken over the long term for the anxiety she has described in the past. You say that you would be willing to have her try one but that the two of you would need to work together to monitor whether the medication is helping. You then ask whether her self-harm has increased and whether she has had a worsening of her suicidal ideation. She answers that she has been self-harming superficially daily rather than a few times a week and continues to have passive suicidal ideation.

4. What do you do next?
    A. Tell her about distress tolerance skills.
    B. Send her to the ER because of an increase in self-harm behavior.
    C. Discuss a schedule for meeting regularly.

Discussion of Options

1=helpful; 2=possibly helpful, continuing reservations; 3=not helpful or even harmful

A. Tell her about distress tolerance skills. [1] This could be a helpful alternative in the short term to cutting and bingeing.
B. Send her to the ER because of an increase in self-harm behavior. [3] This would likely be unhelpful. Jacky's self-harm has escalated in frequency, but it remains superficial and does not require wound care. She also denies any active suicidal ideation.
C. Discuss a schedule for meeting regularly. [1] Jacky is help seeking and has had limited exposure to treatment in the past. She would likely respond well to a lower-intensity generalist approach.

You tell her about distress tolerance skills she can use when she is thinking of self-harming or bingeing and ask whether she would be agreeable to meeting every 2 weeks for 30 minutes. Over time, you help Jacky to make connections between her mood and behaviors. You prescribe an antidepressant for anxiety. You introduce the common interpersonal patterns that unfold for her. She agrees to talk to her parents about her struggles and what you are working on. She receives a call from the psychiatrist for an appointment 6 months after the original referral, but at that point she is doing much better. She goes off to college, and you encourage her to stay in touch.

Vignette 2: Goal Setting and Working With Anger (Jeff)

You are a psychiatry resident working overnight in the ER. Jeff has been brought in by police. He is a 31-year-old male who is currently working bussing tables at a restaurant. He has been feeling "depressed" and then got drunk at a bar, got angry, and ended up in a fistfight. The ER physician consults you because Jeff has had many prior visits to the ER; however, when he is referred to the urgent psychiatry service at discharge, he does not show up to the appointments. He is frustrated that Jeff keeps ending up in the ER and would like you to see him. When Jeff is sober, you interview him and learn that he has a history of mood dysregulation; difficulties controlling his anger (even when sober); difficulties with binge drinking, as well as reckless driving and speeding; and chronic feelings of emptiness. He also describes that he has difficulties being alone and that his relationships usually last only a few months. It is often these breakups that lead to binge drinking and fights. He also becomes quite angry at times with people at work, which has resulted in having to switch jobs frequently. He does not have a history of self-harm or suicidal behavior. He denies any symptoms in keeping with a mood disorder or psychosis.

You have been learning about GPM in your residency program and are required to follow one patient with BPD longitudinally with supervision. You have been looking for a suitable patient and think Jeff might be a good fit. Although he meets criteria for BPD, he does not have a history of suicidal behaviors and has not received basic BPD treatment, so GPM would provide that first step. GPM would help him to make connections between his emotions and behaviors; reduce his anger, aggressive behavior, and binge drinking; and realize some of his work and relationship goals. You also know that in your area of the country, dialectical behavior therapy (DBT) programs require self-harm as a criterion for admission. You provide some psychoeducation to Jeff about BPD, and he is interested in following up with you as an outpatient.

In your first outpatient appointment with Jeff, you review some of the psychoeducation about BPD that you had already discussed in the ER. You then ask Jeff what he would like to be different in his life, and you collaboratively brainstorm treatment goals. He talks about how people he has dated as well as his friends and family are wary of him because of his angry "outbursts." He has never assaulted them but has broken things and punched holes in walls when angry. He has difficulties maintaining relationships, and he binge drinks when relationships end, resulting in bar fights and ER visits. He also notes that he has not been able to keep a job longer than 3 months.

1. What are goals that Jeff could work on that would be in keeping with the GPM model described in this manual?

    A. Explore the problems and benefits associated with drinking in order to decide whether I want to stop binge drinking or not.
    B. Understand where my anger comes from and how it is related to childhood experiences.
    C. Work on the following: 1) express my anger in ways that are more effective; 2) stop binge drinking; 3) maintain employment at the same workplace for at least a year; and 4) have a stable romantic relationship.

Discussion of Options
1=helpful; 2=possibly helpful, continuing reservations; 3=not helpful or even harmful

A. Explore the problems and benefits associated with drinking in order to decide whether I want to stop binge drinking or not. **[2]** Stopping binge drinking would likely be helpful for Jeff, however, he has other difficulties in addition to substance use, including anger behaviors and difficulties in relationship. From a GPM perspective he would likely benefit from having a broader array of behaviorally specific "life worth living" goals.
B. Understand where my anger comes from and how it is related to childhood experiences. **[2]** This goal is more in keeping with an insight-oriented therapeutic approach, such as psychodynamic psychotherapy. This might be helpful to Jeff in the long run; however, it is less likely to result in rapid changes in self-destructive behavior. To be in keeping with the GPM model (or the DBT model), goals need to be behaviorally specific and change needs to be observable and able to be monitored.
C. Work on the following: 1) express my anger in ways that are more effective; 2) stop binge drinking; 3) maintain employment at the same workplace for at least a year; and 4) have a stable romantic relationship. **[1]** These goals are behaviorally specific and can be easily monitored to reflect on whether or not treatment is helpful. These goals are in keeping with the GPM (and DBT) model. In GPM, Jeff would be encouraged to focus on goals 1–3 before focusing on goal 4 because of the principle of "stable work and friendships before love."

Together, the two of you identify goals that are behaviorally specific and that you and Jeff will be able to track in order to know whether treatment is helpful. You discuss why it might make sense to focus on expressing anger effectively, stopping binge drinking, and maintaining employment before working on romantic relationships. You make a framework of your expectations of him and what he can expect from you and agree to meet weekly for the next year if treatment is helping. He understands that you are not able to provide intersession contact and that he is to use a crisis line and the ER in the case of emergency. Jeff also agrees to look into a group available in the community that he could attend and to tell you about this when you meet next week.

At your next session, you introduce the idea of agenda setting so that you can both keep track of what is important to discuss. On your agenda for that day is introducing diary cards and talking about what kind of groups Jeff found in his research over the last week. He would like to talk about an incident at his job yesterday. The two of you agree to first get through some of the practical things, such as group ideas, but to leave time for Jeff to talk about the incident at work. He says that he has found a mindfulness group, which meets down the street from his house, that he would like to attend. It involves some Buddhist teaching but is offered free of charge, which he likes. You provide verbal reinforcement to Jeff for having completed his first homework task by saying, "Sounds like you did a lot of research. I think attending that group will be a helpful part of reaching the goals you set. Good job."

You then introduce the concept of a "diary card." He says that diary cards sound stupid and impractical. "Won't writing about what I do wrong just make things worse? It will make me feel worse thinking about it for sure. Also, I don't want to be carrying around a piece of paper at work all day. That will be embarrassing. This whole thing just seems like busywork."

2. How might you respond?
    A. Validate his concern by saying, "You're right, thinking about the things you want to change might feel crappy in the moment, and it does take some commitment to carry diary cards around and fill them out." Then say, "Never mind, it was only a suggestion. We don't have to do them."
    B. Say, "Well, how about we change the card to make it more convenient for you to have with you at work? What if we only track one behavior?"

C. Validate his concern by saying, "You're right, thinking about the things you want to change might feel crappy in the moment, and it does take some commitment to carry diary cards around and fill them out." Then say, "The reason I think diary cards might be helpful for you is because we will more easily be able to keep track of where you are struggling and where things are improving. Using the diary cards also leaves more time for us during each session because we can review how the previous week went more quickly using the card. Would you be willing to try it for a week and see what you think?"

Discussion of Options

1=helpful; 2=possibly helpful, continuing reservations; 3=not helpful or even harmful

A. Validate his concern by saying, "You're right, thinking about the things you want to change might feel crappy in the moment, and it does take some commitment to carry diary cards around and fill them out." Then say, "Never mind, it was only a suggestion. We don't have to do them." [3] Validating the valid is useful so that the patient feels understood; however, in this situation, if you really think diary cards will be helpful for Jeff, it is a disservice to him not to push for change and highlight why the diary card might be helpful.
B. Say, "Well, how about we change the card to make it more convenient for you to have with you at work? What if we only track one behavior?" [2] Modifying diary cards to be more user-friendly for the patient can be useful; however, it is important to consider how necessary the changes are and what the patient will miss out on with the changes you make. At this point, it might be a bit premature to change the diary card given that Jeff has not yet tried using them.
C. Validate his concern by saying, "You're right, thinking about the things you want to change might feel crappy in the moment, and it does take some commitment to carry diary cards around and fill them out." Then say, "The reason I think diary cards might be helpful for you is because we will more easily be able to keep track of where you are struggling and where things are improving. Using the diary cards also leaves more time for us during each session because we can review more quickly how the previous week went using the card. Would you be willing to try it for a week and see what you think?" [1] With this response, you validate the valid and also push for change by explaining the benefit of the diary card and asking Jeff

to give it a try. This will likely be helpful for the patient if you think using a diary card is of benefit to him.

Jeff reluctantly agrees to try the diary card for a week. You mention that there are "app" versions he might find more convenient at work, or he can fill out the card at the end of each day. You then move on to the incident at work that Jeff had put on the agenda. When you ask him what happened, he says, "My coworker screwed me over, and now my boss is going to know I'm a nut." You say, "Wow, you must be worried. What happened?" He talks about how a coworker asked him in front of his boss what had happened to his eye. He was very embarrassed about having a black eye and paused before coming up with an answer. He chose to say that he got the black eye in a Krav Maga class he went to. Jeff then excused himself from the situation to go to the bathroom and was very angry and punched the cement wall, resulting in his knuckles being cut.

3. What are your next steps?
    A. Do a chain analysis to flesh out the story.
    B. Reinforce the fact that he was skillful to excuse himself and go to the bathroom.
    C. Help him label the emotions he was feeling during the incident.
    D. Offer distress tolerance skills that might help him in moments when he is very angry and might otherwise do something he regrets.
    E. Problem solve with him around what he might do next time.
    F. Introduce opposite action or radical acceptance.

Discussion of Options
1=helpful; 2=possibly helpful, continuing reservations; 3=not helpful or even harmful

A. Do a chain analysis to flesh out the story. **[1]** Jeff's description provides a fair number of links in the chain, but further chain analysis could help to identify additional factors that precipitated the dysregulation.
B. Reinforce the fact that he was skillful to excuse himself and go to the bathroom. **[1]** It is skillful that Jeff was able to excuse himself and go to the washroom rather than yelling at his colleague in front of the boss and making the situation worse. Reinforcing this behavior is important to increase the likelihood that he repeats the behavior in the future.

C. Help him label the emotions he was feeling during the incident. [1] It is likely that Jeff first felt worry about losing his job or being reprimanded when his colleague asked him about his black eye. This fearful response likely then turned into anger toward the colleague. Helping Jeff to identify and label emotions will be an important part of his treatment, as will making connections between those emotions and his behaviors.

D. Offer distress tolerance skills that might help him in moments when he is very angry and might otherwise do something he regrets. [1] Because this is one of your first sessions with Jeff, you could focus closer to the end of the chain and use it as an opportunity for him to use distress tolerance skills as an alternative to punching the wall and injuring himself.

E. Problem solve with him around what he might do next time. [1] Problem solving around what Jeff can do when he is angry at work in the future and then having him try this as homework might be useful.

F. Introduce opposite action or radical acceptance. [2] Opposite action and radical acceptance could be useful in this situation and could be described at this juncture. However, because these techniques can be challenging for patients to learn and implement, they could be introduced a bit later after Jeff first has a handle on some of the distress tolerance skills.

You decide that Jeff's description provided a sufficient chain and focus on teaching him one distress tolerance skill that he can use the next time he is overwhelmed by anger. You then problem solve with him around how he could go about using this distress tolerance skill at work and troubleshoot any difficulties he might run into. You ask him to try and fill out the diary card between now and next week and to try practicing the distress tolerance skill when he is not distressed at least three times before next week so he is familiar with it and can use it when needed.

Later that week, you meet with your supervisor, Dr. Lee, who asks you about your formulation of Jeff's behavior from an interpersonal hypersensitivity perspective. You say that it seems that when Jeff perceives the threat that he is going to be rejected (e.g., his boss finding out he got a black eye from a barroom fight), he becomes fearful and then angry toward others (e.g., his coworker and himself). Jeff then copes by expressing his anger physically (e.g., punching walls). In this most recent incident with his boss, he was not actually rejected (he kept his job, and there were no consequences), and the anger/fear then dissipated. In other situations where he is actually rejected, he becomes more impulsive and binge drinks, resulting in barroom fights. He is then sent to the ER by the police, and in this contained environment, he returns to baseline.

Dr. Lee says, "It is not unlikely that at some point you will screw up in some way or something will happen and Jeff will feel rejected by you. Given his past history of difficulties with anger toward coworkers, I suspect he might at some point become angry with you, too. How will you respond to that?"

4. How will you respond to Jeff when he inevitably expresses anger toward you?
   A. Validate the valid by saying, "I get that you're angry right now because I'm late. Anyone would be."
   B. Offer distress tolerance skills to decrease anger in the moment. "I see that you're very angry right now. Would you mind if we do some distress tolerance skills to bring the anger down so we can figure this out?"
   C. Inquire about why he is angry. "I get the sense that you're really angry right now. What's up?"
   D. Highlight how this might fit the interpersonal pattern he seems to fall into by saying, "I get the sense that you're really angry with me right now. I wonder if that is because I said I can't stay late and that felt like a rejection."

Discussion of Options
1=helpful; 2=possibly helpful, continuing reservations; 3=not helpful or even harmful

A. Validate the valid by saying, "I get that you're angry right now because I'm late. Anyone would be." **[1]** Validation is a good way to diffuse anger. However, it is important to validate only the aspects of the situation that are valid.
B. Offer distress tolerance skills to decrease anger in the moment. "I see that you're very angry right now. Would you mind if we do some distress tolerance skills to bring the anger down so we can figure this out?" **[1]** If someone is very angry, distress tolerance skills can sometimes help. Note that it can be helpful to express validation first before offering distress tolerance skills.
C. Inquire about why he is angry by saying, "I get the sense that you're really angry right now. What's up?" **[2]** This can be helpful, but it might lead to more difficulty if the person is so angry their brain has

gone "offline." If the person is very dysregulated, it might be best to help the person get closer to their baseline using validation and/or distress tolerance skills before asking them to reflect.

D. Highlight how this might fit the interpersonal pattern he seems to fall into. "I get the sense that you're really angry with me right now. I wonder if that is because I said I can't stay late and that felt like a rejection." [2] This discussion might be useful in the long term, but similar to option C, it is unlikely that the person will be able to reflect in a complex way when they are very dysregulated. Using validation and skills to get their brain back "online" is the first step.

You find Dr. Lee's supervision very helpful, and you continue to work with Jeff to find ways for him to express himself more effectively, reduce unwanted behaviors, and be more mindful of the primary emotions underlying his anger (which turn out to be mainly fear in situations where he is likely to be rejected). After a month of working together, you and he are starting to get a sense of some of his common patterns, and he has increased awareness when they are occurring. He agrees to remove alcohol from his apartment, at least temporarily, to reduce the chance that he will binge drink when emotionally dysregulated.

By the end of 6 months, Jeff is no longer acting out physically when he is angry and has not had any further drinking binges or fights. He also has taken on a new project at work and is very busy. The two of you have also worked in sessions on building up friendships, and Jeff has joined a social sports club. You discuss whether it would be in his best interest to meet every second week rather than weekly given how busy he is, and he agrees. You see him biweekly for the next 6 months and then monthly for the following 6 months. He continues to work at the same company and starts dating. After working together for a year and a half, you and Jeff both agree that he is doing much better and agree to end your therapy together.

Vignette 3: Good Psychiatric Management Follow-Up After Standard Dialectical Behavior Therapy (Suzanne)

You are a case worker at a community health agency. You have been asked to see Suzanne, who was taken to the ER 2 days ago with a serious overdose. Suzanne is a 41-year-old female who lives in subsidized housing and has two cats. She worked at a grocery store in her 20s but has been supported by disability payments since then. In her chart, you read that she has previously been diagnosed with BPD and attended a standard DBT program 3 months ago, where she did very well. She went from being admitted to the hospital several times a year for suicide attempts to having no suicide attempts while she was in the program. Unfortunately, since she completed the program 3 months ago, she has been admitted to the hospital twice with serious overdoses. She has also been overdosing several times a week on cough syrup, which is problematic because she has a history of liver damage. She has had difficulties keeping a job and making friends and is isolated. Her overdoses tend to follow negative social interactions with her mother, who lives in the same building as Suzanne does. She also sometimes has negative social interactions with the housing committee in her building. When you meet with Suzanne, she is no longer suicidal and is able to identify that she overdosed following a fight with her mother, after which Suzanne was sitting in her apartment feeling very alone and thinking about how things were never going to get better.

1. Given what you know about Suzanne so far, what might be a helpful treatment approach?
    A. It sounds like she did very well in DBT. Continuing to work with her around using skills to stop overdosing would likely be useful.
    B. It might be that Suzanne relapsed after discharge because she had not yet built much of a network outside of treatment. Focusing on work and friendships outside of treatment might be helpful.
    C. Suzanne has already had standard DBT, an intensive specialized treatment. She is unlikely to be helped by further treatment.

Discussion of Options

1=helpful; 2=possibly helpful, continuing reservations; 3=not helpful or even harmful

A. It sounds like she did very well in DBT. Continuing to work with her around using skills to stop overdosing would likely be useful. [2] This could be helpful. However, it would be important to identify what changed for Suzanne after treatment ended to prevent something similar from happening when your treatment with her ends.
B. It might be that Suzanne relapsed after discharge because she had not yet built much of a network outside of treatment. Focusing on work and friendships outside of treatment might be helpful. [1] It sounds as though Suzanne did very well in DBT but was unable to increase

her engagement in friendships and to work significantly during the 1-year time frame of treatment. Continuing to work on building this network might reduce relapse when she is not being followed by a clinician. The long-standing course and severity of her illness might mean that she requires more time to build a "life worth living."

C. Suzanne has already had standard DBT, an intensive specialized treatment. She is unlikely to be helped by further treatment. **[3]** Suzanne responded well to DBT. She might respond to further treatment using a GPM model, especially if part of what she needs to work on is building a social network and becoming more independent.

When you meet with Suzanne, she is able to clearly describe what she learned in DBT and why she found it helpful. She reports that when the program ended, she realized she was just going back to the "same old shit." Without her clinician and other group members to talk to, she had only her mother for support. She and her clinician had worked on her goal of making friends and meeting more people, but this happened late in treatment and she says she stopped working on it after treatment ended. She has not overdosed since her last visit to the ER when she was referred to you. In the meeting, Suzanne looks somewhat hopeless and says, "I don't think you can help me. My last therapist was great, and I'm still right back where I started."

2. What do you say?

A. "You're right, the case is hopeless!"

B. "Well, why don't we list the pros and cons of your choosing to work with me or not?"

C. "If you don't want to work with me, that's no problem; it's your choice. It is likely that you will continue having unpleasant interactions with your mom and overdosing frequently. It is really up to you, though. I have no interest in forcing you to do a treatment you're not interested in."

D. "I can understand that it would be hard to start a new treatment given how hard you have already worked in your last treatment and the way things have been since you ended treatment. I also think that working together could be quite helpful so that you can continue building on what you have already started."

Discussion of Options

1=helpful; 2=possibly helpful, continuing reservations; 3=not helpful or even harmful

A. "You're right, the case is hopeless!" [2] Making an irreverent statement is in keeping with both GPM and DBT. In this case, however, it might not be the best approach given the scenario described. If Suzanne's hopelessness were very prominent or repetitive, an irreverent statement might shake things up, but in this case, simple validation would be sufficient.

B. "Well, why don't we list the pros and cons of your choosing to work with me or not?" [2] Evaluating pros and cons can be a strategy to strengthen and evaluate a commitment someone has made. Given that Suzanne has experience with DBT, she is likely familiar with considering pros and cons, so this might be a strategy she could jump into. At the same time, given the scenario, suggesting pros and cons right away might seem a bit jarring without exploring the issue a little bit first.

C. "If you don't want to work with me, that's no problem; it's your choice. It is likely that you will continue having unpleasant interactions with your mom and overdosing frequently. It is really up to you, though. I have no interest in forcing you to do a treatment you're not interested in." [2] This is an example of "freedom to choose" in that you are highlighting that treatment is a choice but also pointing out that the alternative is bleak. Like the technique of irreverence, this type of strategy might be more helpful when a patient is more fixed on a certain outcome.

D. "I can understand that it would be hard to start a new treatment given how hard you have already worked in your last treatment and the way things have been since you ended treatment. I also think that working together could be quite helpful so that you can continue building on what you have already started." [1] This response balances acceptance and change. It might be enough to help Suzanne get "wise mind" back online. If she continues to become more hopeless, then the responses described in options A and C would become helpful.

Suzanne agrees to see you every 2 weeks for up to 1 year to work on her goal of building friendships. You also encourage her to pursue a productive activity such as volunteering or work, and she agrees to this. You make a safety plan, and she understands that you are not able to provide intersession contact and that she is to use a crisis line and the ER in the case of emergency. You also encourage her mom's involvement in treatment given that Suzanne's overdoses are often preceded by arguments with her mother. Suzanne is reluctant and says, "My mom wouldn't get it. She thinks this is all just a bunch of psychobabble." Over the next month, Suzanne does quite well. You offer to see her for an extra session to help her prepare her resumé to apply for jobs. She gets a part-time job at a dog daycare business, which she enjoys. She adjusts her hours so she is able to maintain her disability and drug payments. As homework, she begins brainstorming about clubs she can join and other ways she can expand her social network.

At your next appointment, Suzanne is extremely distressed. She and her mom got into an argument a few days earlier. Suzanne's mom told her that her job with the dogs was silly and below her capacity. After Suzanne stormed out of her mom's apartment, her mom was upset and stopped taking her "water pills" for a few days and ended up with worsening heart failure. Her mom was admitted to the hospital last night. Suzanne says she herself is suicidal and "can't handle it." She says, "I need to be admitted to the hospital or I am going to kill myself, for real this time."

3. How do you respond?

   A. Call the police to take her to the ER for a psychiatric assessment and inpatient admission.
   B. Encourage her to use skills to reduce her distress so she is able to use "wise mind" regarding whether hospitalization is the most effective option for her.
   C. Say to her, "I don't think hospitalization is the best idea because you will lose your job with the dogs that you really enjoy and our work together will be put on hold. At the same time, I'm worried that if I don't hospitalize you, you will overdose. What do you think I should do?"

Discussion of Options

1=helpful; 2=possibly helpful, continuing reservations; 3=not helpful or even harmful

A. Call the police to take her to the ER for a psychiatric assessment and inpatient admission. **[2]** This may be necessary, but hospitalization should be avoided if possible because Suzanne will not be able to work on "building a life" while she is in the hospital.
B. Encourage her to use skills to reduce her distress so she is able to use "wise mind" regarding whether hospitalization is the most effective option for her. **[1]** Given Suzanne's level of distress, this might be a good option so that you can have a more productive discussion about hospitalization and alternatives.

C. Say to her, "I don't think hospitalization is the best idea because you will lose your job with the dogs that you really enjoy and our work together will be put on hold. At the same time, I'm worried that if I don't hospitalize you, you will overdose. What do you think I should do?" [1] If Suzanne is in a space where her brain is online, presenting her with this dilemma and leaving it in her court is a good option. Depending on her level of distress, doing distress tolerance or emotion regulation skills before having this discussion might be helpful.

Suzanne is able to use paced breathing paired with progressive muscle relaxation to reduce her autonomic arousal. She is then able to think more clearly about the dilemma that you present to her about hospitalization. She wants to try to avoid hospitalization so she does not lose her job. She is able to problem solve with you around how she can keep herself safe until your next appointment. She remains reluctant to involve her mom in her treatment, but you are insistent about this because of the role their relationship plays in Suzanne's suicide attempts.

After resuming her diuretic, Suzanne's mother is released from the hospital. You and Suzanne plan how you will approach a meeting with her mother. The plan is for you to provide some psychoeducation to Suzanne's mother about BPD and explain your work together and then allow her mother to ask any questions and explain any worries she has. Suzanne's mother agrees to accompany Suzanne to her next appointment. She appears quite guarded at first and makes several critical comments about Suzanne but then starts to open up when you validate some of the valid things she says. You continue to meet with Suzanne and her mother jointly at some of your appointments, and Suzanne works with some of the skills she learned in DBT to be more interpersonally effective with her mother. Suzanne continues to work at the dog daycare and joins a crocheting group where she makes two friends and several acquaintances. You start meeting monthly after Suzanne has been seeing you for around 6 months because your sessions begin to interfere with her work and social schedule. When you have been working together for almost a year, Suzanne starts volunteering at a dog shelter in addition to working at the dog daycare, and the two of you agree to end treatment given her busy schedule.

Vignette 4: Medication Management (Kiran)

Kiran is a 20-year old female who currently works as a receptionist at a law office. She was referred from the ER to a 3-month DBT skills group.

She has not had prior BPD-focused treatment, and the ER physician felt that less intensive treatment now could curb the progression of clinical severity and preserve and improve Kiran's functioning. You are a general psychiatrist and have agreed to see her twice a month while she is in the group. You have recently read about GPM and are looking forward to using this approach with Kiran.

In your first consultation with Kiran, she appears to have a clear history of social anxiety in addition to BPD. Kiran is feeling very anxious about attending the group and, as a result, has been taking more of her medications than she is supposed to. You learn that she is currently taking quetiapine and lorazepam. She asks for a medication to help with her BPD.

1. How do you respond?

A. Tell her that quetiapine and lorazepam are not the best options for social anxiety, and advise her that she should stop taking them and start an SSRI.

B. Explain to her that medications are not helpful for BPD and that you should work together to taper the medications she is currently taking.

C. Inquire about how helpful her current medications are. Provide some psychoeducation about BPD and medication response in patients with BPD. Also, provide psychoeducation about treating specific symptoms and comorbidities, as well as the importance of monitoring for improvement.

Discussion of Options
1=helpful; 2=possibly helpful, continuing reservations; 3=not helpful or even harmful

A. Tell her that quetiapine and lorazepam are not the best options for social anxiety, and advise her that she should stop taking them and start an SSRI. [2] This is true; however, it is also important to learn more about the Kiran's experience with the medications she is taking and what has been helpful or not helpful about them. A curious and collaborative approach can go a long way toward more productive medication management.

B. Explain to her that medications are not helpful for BPD and that you should work together to taper the medications she is currently taking. [2] It may be useful to taper the medications Kiran is taking; however, the situation is more nuanced. She also needs to be aware that comorbidities can sometimes be ameliorated with medications and that medication also has a limited role in targeting certain symptoms of BPD.

C. Inquire about how helpful her current medications are. Provide some psychoeducation about BPD and medication response in patients with BPD. Also, provide psychoeducation about treating specific symptoms and comorbidities, as well as the importance of monitoring for improvement. [1] Having this detailed discussion with Kiran from the outset can save much grief in the long term by helping to avoid multiple medication trials and polypharmacy.

You speak to Kiran about the fact that there are no medications that "treat BPD" and tell her that the group she is attending is likely to offer more improvement than a medication will. You say that treating other conditions, such as social anxiety, can help her to get the most out of the group. You ask Kiran how she thinks her current medications are helping her. She says she has not noticed much of a difference with the quetiapine but finds the lorazepam helpful in moments when she is very anxious. You discuss how lorazepam can be helpful in the moment but is less helpful in the long term. You suggest that Kiran would likely benefit from an SSRI to target social anxiety, and she agrees to try that. You suggest that it might be best to taper her quetiapine before starting a new medication to have more clarity about what is helpful. You suggest tapering the lorazepam over time. You talk to her about how important it is to monitor for tangible markers of improvement with the SSRI medication to determine whether it is helping and warn her that it will likely take at least 2 weeks to start working and 4–6 weeks to have full effect.

As you continue to follow Kiran for medication management and she attends the group, she stops overdosing and self-harming. The quetiapine is stopped, and her lorazepam is tapered over time. She finds the SSRI helpful for social anxiety, and the two of you have monitored what is helpful about the medication: specifically, she is now able to talk to strangers more easily at parties, speak to her boss when needed at work, and use public washrooms when other people are present.

In your sessions with Kiran, she describes herself as a "chameleon" and says that she remains unsure of "who she is" and acts very differently with different groups of people. She also describes not feeling fulfilled in her job as a receptionist but not knowing what to do next.

2. What would you suggest?
   A. These issues will be addressed in the DBT skills group when the group works on identifying individuals' values. You should continue to focus only on medication management.

B. If Kiran is interested, you could have her work on her autobiography as homework in between your appointments.
C. You are involved in medication management only. To avoid splitting, you should remain focused only on medication management.
D. You could work with Kiran on identifying her goals and values.

Discussion of Options

1=helpful; 2=possibly helpful, continuing reservations; 3=not helpful or even harmful

A. These issues will be addressed in the DBT skills group when the group works on identifying individuals'. values. You should continue to focus only on medication management. **[2]** Some of Kiran's difficulties around "sense of self" will likely be addressed in the DBT group. However, providing additional individual guidance to Kiran would not be harmful and would likely be helpful.
B. If Kiran is interested, you could have her work on her autobiography as homework in between your sessions. **[1]** If Kiran has the time, in addition to her other homework from the DBT group, working on her autobiography could be useful to help her develop a more coherent narrative. It may be useful for you, Kiran, and the group leaders to discuss whether this would interfere at all with Kiran's progress in the group.
C. You are involved in medication management only. To avoid splitting, you should remain focused only on medication management. **[3]** If there is open communication between you, the group leaders, and Kiran, it is unlikely to be problematic if you work with her on certain therapeutic tasks concurrent to the group.
D. You could work with Kiran on identifying her goals and values. **[1]** Similar to working on her autobiography, working with Kiran on identifying her goals and values would provide a sense of direction that can bolster a sense of identity.

Kiran feels that the group members have worked enough on identifying their goals and values in the DBT group, but she is very interested in the idea of working on her autobiography. Although you make it clear that this would be extra homework in addition to what she is working on for skills group, she remains interested. At her next medication visit, you start out by asking Kiran to draw her family tree and explain it to you. For the next appointment, you ask her to make a timeline with significant events in her life and explain it to you. She says that she found writing the timeline to be an interesting experience and that it really put things into perspective for her.

As the group comes to a close, Kiran remains interested in writing out a more detailed narrative. You will no longer be following up with her after group sessions end, and you suggest that she continue the autobiography and share it with certain family members and friends. You end treatment with Kiran, and her family doctor resumes managing her prescriptions. A year later, you hear from Kiran. She sends you a thank you card to let you know she is doing well and has been studying to be a paralegal and plans to begin working in that field after graduation.

8

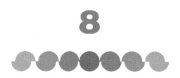

Conclusion

Anne K.I. Sonley, J.D., M.D., FRCPC

Lois W. Choi-Kain, M.D., M.Ed.

This manual draws from good psychiatric management (GPM), integrating principles derived from dialectical behavior therapy (DBT), to extend the reach of good evidence-based care for borderline personality disorder (BPD). GPM is an approach to treating BPD that requires minimal training, is flexible, and is feasible for generalists to learn and use. DBT is the most well-studied BPD treatment and one of the most popular BPD treatments in North America and around the world. All mental health clinicians, even if they are not specialists trained in providing DBT, are likely to benefit from having an understanding of what DBT is and when a patient might require DBT and from being able to use select DBT strategies. Our hope is that this manual provides generalist mental health clinicians with a brief overview of what GPM and DBT are, as well as guidance on how a generalist might provide GPM informed by DBT principles.

In summary, three of the most important things a mental health clinician can do when treating patients with BPD is to provide them with psychoeducation about the disorder, help them set goals around building a "life worth living," and help them make connections between emotions, thoughts, and behaviors. Both DBT and GPM encourage clinicians to discuss the BPD diagnosis with patients. Providing psychoeducation about the etiology, treatment, and prognosis of BPD has been shown, on its own, to lead to symptom improvement in people with BPD (Zanarini and Frankenburg 2008, Zanarini et al. 2018). In terms of etiology, GPM proposes that people with BPD are naturally more interpersonally sensitive and that it is often incidents of interpersonal rejection or hostility that prompt the manifestation of BPD symptoms (e.g., self-harm, anger, substance use and other impulsive behaviors, suicidal behavior). DBT proposes that people with BPD are naturally more emotionally intense and that a combination of repeated invalidation of their emotions and lack of skills for managing emotional intensity is what leads to BPD symptoms. These two theories of BPD are complementary, and it can be useful to explain both to patients to broaden the tools they have for understanding and managing their symptoms.

Both DBT and GPM highlight that the main goal when treating BPD is collaborating with the patient to build a life worth living. Stopping self-harm, substance use, disordered eating, or other problematic behaviors is viewed as an important step toward building a life worth living. Whether the clinician is meeting with a patient for a one-time medication consult or following a patient for a long time, collaborating with the patient to develop life-worth-living goals can provide a focus for treatment.

After goals of treatment have been identified, a key strategy in all effective treatments for BPD is to help patients make connections between current life events and their emotions, thoughts, and behaviors. In both DBT and GPM, self-harm and impulsive behaviors are viewed as coping mechanisms that occur in the context of emotional distress and interpersonal rejection. It is important for clinicians to work with patients to identify common patterns that lead to self-harm and other impulsive behaviors and to determine the function of these behaviors. Chain analysis can be a useful strategy for making these connections. It is important for a clinician and patient to make a plan for alternative coping strategies that the patient can use when distressed. In general, the current problems of day-to-day living are the main focus of DBT and GPM sessions. Clinicians are active in sessions and encourage patients to collaborate as active participants.

In addition to providing clinicians with guidance on how to approach the "what" of treating BPD (providing psychoeducation, collaborative goal setting, and helping the patient make connections between emotions, thoughts, and behaviors), DBT and GPM also give guidance about the "how" of treating BPD. When treating people with BPD, clinicians need to be open and direct about their own thought processes. Most patients with BPD have had invalidating and traumatic experiences in childhood and understandably may not be very trusting of other people, including clinicians. By being open and direct about their own thought processes, clinicians can help increase trust between themselves and their patients. Providing validation is another way to increase openness and trust and can also reduce patients' emotion dysregulation. Both GPM and DBT also highlight that self-disclosure within personal limits can be a useful teaching tool and that brief irreverent or humorous statements can be used to gently nudge patients "off balance" when they are particularly stuck or hopeless.

Another "how" of treating BPD common to both GPM and DBT is using a structured approach. When a clinician is beginning to work with a patient with BPD, it can be useful to discuss treatment duration and frequency at the first meeting and to highlight that treatment will continue only if it proves to be helpful. Treatment contracts can be used to outline clinician and patient expectations and to provide guidelines for treatment. There will likely be times when both the clinician and the patient will step outside of the framework, and having a framework provides a cue to discuss these deviations and to help get the treatment back on track. Similarly, having a consistent structured approach to follow within sessions creates consistency and predictability for both clinician and patient.

Both DBT and GPM make recommendations around intersession contact with patients. Intersession contact supports patients as they find new ways to cope in crisis situations. In GPM, intersession availability depends on the clinician's limits and should be discussed with the patient in advance. It is important to highlight to a patient that relying on the therapist as the main way to prevent suicide is not feasible. Misuse of intersession contact is rare, and when it occurs, it is addressed at the next session.

Standard DBT involves a group component, and in GPM, patient participation in any type of structured group—a DBT skills group, interpersonal group, support group, or a drug or alcohol recovery group, among other possibilities—is highly recommended. When a patient is involved in a group or is seeing multiple treaters, it is important for all treaters involved to maintain open communication. If a patient is frustrated with a treater, it is important for the treater to tolerate this and validate what is valid about the patient's concerns. It is also important to avoid vilification of other treaters. It can be helpful to have the patient involved in communication between treaters to increase transparency and to encourage the patient to self-advocate. Finally, having weekly clinician-to-clinician support is an important part of DBT, and having clinician supervision in some form is also strongly recommended in GPM.

Despite the many commonalities between the approaches to treating BPD outlined in DBT and GPM, each approach has certain useful strategies that are unique to that approach. The DBT-specific strategies highlighted in this manual include dialectics (acceptance and change), commitment strategies, approach to treatment-interfering behavior, diary cards and agenda setting, and a summary of 10 key DBT skills. The GPM-specific strategies highlighted include treatment response timelines, approaches to treating comorbidities, psychopharmacology, involvement of significant others, focus on interpersonal dynamics, drafting of an autobiography, and focus on function.

We hope this guide has been helpful for generalists—including family doctors, social workers, psychotherapists, general psychiatrists, psychiatry residents, psychologists, psychiatric nurses, and all other mental health clinicians—who assess, treat, or follow people with BPD. If you are interested in further training in GPM, there are now free online continuing education modules available through Harvard Medical School Continuing Medical Education (see appendix E for further details). We welcome any feedback you might have about what works in your applications of GPM and DBT and where additional tools or guidance may be helpful. We believe in your ability to make use of what we have shared with you to establish productive and meaningful relationships with many patients who suffer from the problems of BPD. You might help many patients change their lives. As the late John Gunderson said, "You don't need to be a specialist, to be selflessly devoted, or to have a larger-than-life personality to be 'good enough'; you do need to be warm, reliable, interested, and unintimidated" (Gunderson and Links 2014, pp. 3–4).

References

Gunderson JG, Links P: Handbook of Good Psychiatric Management for Borderline Personality Disorder. Washington, DC, American Psychiatric Publishing, 2014

Zanarini MC, Frankenburg FR: A preliminary, randomized trial of psychoeducation for women with borderline personality disorder. J Pers Disord 22(3):284–90, 2008

Zanarini MC, Conkey LC, Temes CM, Fitzmaurice G: Randomized controlled trial of web-based psychoeducation for women with borderline personality disorder. J Clin Psychiatry 79(3), 2018

Common Values

In both DBT and GPM, patients are encouraged to identify their values and goals with respect to what constitutes a life worth living. It can be difficult for people to identify what their values are given that "an unstable sense of self" is one of the symptoms of BPD. Sometimes it can be helpful to provide patients with a list of common values and to ask them to rank-order the values in terms of their importance.

Schwartz (1992, 2012) has identified certain values that seem to be common across cultures that can be a useful starting place for helping patients identify their own values. These values include the following elements:

- Being self-directed and independent
- Creativity
- Exploration
- Curiosity
- Privacy
- Excitement and new experiences
- Pleasure and enjoyment
- Social approval or recognition
- Reliability
- Integrity
- Maintaining traditions
- Attending to relationships
- Contributing to the larger community
- Being open to understanding different people's perspectives or experience
- Achieving things, performance, and success

- Being powerful and able to influence others
- Being wealthy
- Working at self-development
- Security, stability
- Health
- Cleanliness
- Behaving respectfully, politeness
- Self-restraint, self-discipline
- Spirituality
- Being part of a group
- Helping or caring for others
- Promoting social justice, equality
- Caring for nature and the environment

References

Schwartz SH: Universals in the content and structure of values: theory and empirical tests in 20 countries, in Advances in Experimental Social Psychology, Vol 25. Edited by Zanna M. New York, Academic Press, 1992, pp 1–65

Schwartz SH: An overview of the Schwartz theory of basic values. Online Readings in Psychology and Culture 2(1), 2012

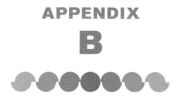

Sample Treatment Agreement

Patient's Agreement

I commit to treatment for the next 6 months. I agree to meet every week for 50 minutes and to arrive on time for my appointments. I commit to canceling 2 weeks in advance if I am going to be away. I will be charged $20 for each missed appointment if I do not give 2 weeks advance notice. If I miss four sessions in a row, I will be out of treatment. I agree not to end my life during treatment and to follow the plan my clinician and I have come up with if I have strong suicidal urges. I give my clinician permission to contact the people listed on my crisis plan in the case of an emergency or if I am at risk of dropping out of treatment. I agree to keep my BMI at 18 or above so I am able to engage in treatment, and I agree not to come to sessions intoxicated. I agree to engage in work, studies, or a volunteer commitment by the time I am 3 months into treatment.

Clinician's Agreement

I agree to be available by phone or email from the hours of 9 A.M.–5 P.M. Monday through Friday. Outside of those hours, please use the crisis plan we have developed. I commit to including you in discussions I have with other treatment providers whenever possible and to include you in discussions with family members or significant others.

_____   _____
Patient Signature   Date

_____   _____
Clinician Signature   Date

Sample Crisis Plan

Background information

Past attempts	2008 overdose on 20 quetiapine, 2017 overdose on bottle of Tylenol requiring admission to intensive care unit
Self-harm	Daily superficial cutting (not requiring medical attention)
Common precipitants	Break-up with partner, feeling rejected
Warning signs	Not attending classes, increased alcohol use
Reinforcing factors	Ex-boyfriends have come to visit at the hospital
Reasons for not self-harming	Scars, distressing for past boyfriends
Reasons for not killing yourself	Not hurting grandmother
Reasons for living	Things might get better someday, finishing degree
Current medications	Sertraline 200 mg daily, dispensed monthly
Emergency contacts	Mom (___) ___-___, sister (___) ___-___

Distress tolerance plan

Step 1: Use my helpful distress tolerance strategies.

Use ice, intense exercise, paced breathing, distraction (e.g., watching a funny movie, petting cat, walking dog, playing Sudoku, doing yoga, taking a bath, eating popcorn)

Step 2: Contact supportive people.

Helpful: friend Sarah (___) ___-____ and friend Erin (___) ___-____
Not helpful: mom or sister

Step 3: Contact my clinician.

Phone: (___) ___-____ or email clinician@clinician.com

Step 4: Call crisis line.

Phone: (___) ___-____

Step 5: Go to emergency room.

Address: General Hospital, 123 Hospital Street

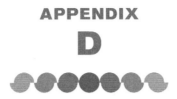

Sample Diary Card

The diary card contains a quick overview of how things were for the patient over the previous week. Patients are expected to monitor their behaviors daily on these cards. The cards should be personalized to the individual patient so that the behaviors tracked are relevant.

Sample diary card (Med=medication; SI=suicidal ideation)

Day	Date	Self-Harm (Urge) 0–5	Self-Harm (Behav)	SI (Urge) 0–5	SI (Behav)	Alcohol (Urge) 0–5	Alcohol (Behav)	Drugs (Urge) 0–5	Drugs (Behav)	Med Misuse (Urge) 0–5	Med Misuse (Behav)	Binge (Urge) 0–5	Binge (Behav)	Sadness 0–5	Fear 0–5	Anger 0–5	Shame 0–5	Joy 0–5
M																		
T																		
W																		
T																		
F																		
S																		
S																		

Sample diary card as filled in by patient (Med=medication; SI=suicidal ideation)

Day	Date	Self-Harm (Urge) 0–5	Self-Harm (Behav)	SI (Urge) 0–5	SI (Behav)	Alcohol (Urge) 0–5	Alcohol (Behav)	Drugs (Urge) 0–5	Drugs (Behav)	Med Misuse (Urge) 0–5	Med Misuse (Behav)	Binge (Urge) 0–5	Binge (Behav)	Sadness 0–5	Fear 0–5	Anger 0–5	Shame 0–5	Joy 0–5
M	Aug 10	1	0	0	0	0	0	0	0	0	0	3	0	2	2	3	3	4
T	Aug 11	2	0	0	0	0	0	0	0	0	0	3	0	1	4	2	3	0
W	Aug 12	2	0	0	0	0	0	0	0	0	0	5	X	1	3	2	3	0
T	Aug 13	3	0	3	0	3	0	2	0	0	0	5	X	2	3	1	3	0
F	Aug 14	2	0	0	0	3	X	3	X	0	0	5	X	4	2	3	4	0
S	Aug 15	5	X	5	0	5	X	5	X	0	0	5	X	5	5	5	5	0
S	Aug 16	5	0	4	0	2	0	2	0	0	0	2	0	3	4	3	5	0

Free Online Good Psychiatric Management Training

McLean Hospital's Gunderson Personality Disorders Institute offers continuing education training in good psychiatric management (GPM) through Harvard Medical School Continuing Medical Education (HMS CME) online (http://hms.harvard.edu/BPD). GPM, an empirically supported treatment approach, has been demonstrated to match the effectiveness of dialectical behavior therapy in treating patients with borderline personality disorder (McMain et al. 2009). The course—offered for free until 2022—teaches mental health professionals and primary care clinicians what they need to know to become competent providers who can derive satisfaction from treating these patients. CME credits are available for physicians, psychologists, social workers, licensed mental health counselors, and nurses.

Through lectures, case illustrations, and interactive decision points, the course covers management strategies that incorporate practicality, good sense, and flexibility. Techniques and interventions that facilitate the patient's trust and willingness to become a proactive collaborator are described. The course reviews guidelines for handling the common and usually most burdensome issues of managing suicidality and self-harm (e.g., intersession crises, threats as a call for help, excessive use of emergency departments or hospitals). In addition, it describes how and when psychiatrists can usefully integrate group, family, or other psychotherapies.

Reference

McMain SF, Links PS, Gnam WH, et al: A randomized trial of dialectical behavior therapy versus general psychiatric management for borderline personality disorder. Am J Psychiatry 166(12):1365–1374, 2009

Index

*Page numbers printed in **boldface** type refer to tables or figures.*